Children and Grief

CHILDREN AND GRIEF

When a Parent Dies

J. WILLIAM WORDEN

THE GUILFORD PRESS
New York   London

© 1996 J. William Worden
Published by the Guilford Press
A Division of Guilford Publications, Inc.
72 Spring Street, New York, NY 10012

Printed in the United States of America

This book is printed on acid-free paper.

Last digit is print number: 9   8   7   6   5   4   3   2   1

Library of Congress Cataloging-in-Publication Data
Worden, J. William (James William)
    Children and grief : when a parent dies / J. William Worden.
      p. cm.
    Includes bibliographical references and index.
    ISBN 1-57230-148-1
    1. Bereavement in children.   2. Parents—Death—Psychological
aspects.   3. Grief in children.   4. Children and death.   I. Title.
BF723.G75W67   1996
155.9'37'083—dc20   96-29010
                                    CIP

*To the children and parents
in the Child Bereavement Study
who allowed us to see
their pain and their triumphs*

Acknowledgments

There are many people who contributed to my thinking and to the ideas presented in the book. First and foremost I want to thank my two principal colleagues on the Child Bereavement Study, Drs. Phyllis Silverman and Steven Nickman. Dr. Silverman is truly one of the pioneers in the study of grief and bereavement. Her seminal work on widows and self-help groups, begun while she was at Harvard's Laboratory of Community Psychiatry, has set the tone for most of the intervention with the conjugally bereaved around the world today. Dr. Nickman, child psychiatrist on our study, has had a long-time professional interest in children's adaptation to loss and separation. His work on adoptive families is well known.

We were fortunate to have had a cadre of experienced professionals on our interviewing staff. These included Jane Allen, Susan Creditor, Diane D'Alessio, Hadley Fisk, Jane Lynch, Paul Lynch, Alyn Roberson, Rebecca Starr, and Marilyn Weller. We are grateful to them for the sensitive way they were able to interview the children and surviving parents.

Consulting to the study were Drs. Robert Harrison, Blythe Clinche, Deborah Walker, and Theodore Colton. They helped us formulate the ideas and assessments used in the study.

Assisting with the data management and analysis were Drs. Naji Abi-Hashem and Robert Horon and Mr. Douglas Herr. Their contributions are gratefully acknowledged.

Funding for the Child Bereavement Study was provided by grants from the National Institute of Mental Health (MH-41791), the National Funeral Directors Association, and the Hillenbrand

Corporation. Without this generous funding a longitudinal study would have been impossible.

Editorial assistance was provided by Barbara Watkins and Rochelle Serwator of The Guilford Press, Marilyn Weller, Pat Worden, and Karin Worden.

Thanks go to Betty Davies and Darlene McCowan, who shared research data and ideas on the comparison of sibling loss and parental loss.

Dr. Edwin Cassem, Chief of Psychiatry at the Massachusetts General Hospital, and Dr. Keith Edwards, Dean of the Rosemead School of Psychology in California, gave time and encouragement to this project.

A special appreciation goes to the bereaved families who allowed us to come into their lives at a tender time and who candidly shared with us the experience of loss. It is to all of them that this book is dedicated.

Contents

THREE
HOW WE CAN HELP BEREAVED CHILDREN

Children and Grief

Introduction

Although there have been many books written on bereaved children, few are based on studies that give us definitive information on this population. The research findings on childhood grief are often inconsistent and differ among studies. This general lack of consensus is due, in part, to several serious methodological limitations. First, some studies fail to use a demographically matched nonbereaved control group (Felner et al., 1981; Kaffman & Elizur, 1983). Without this, one cannot say whether the observed behavior is due to bereavement or due to age, gender, or developmental differences. A second limitation is the use of different measures to assess psychological problems (Kaffman & Elizur, 1983; Van Eerdewegh et al., 1982). A lack of standardized assessment makes it difficult, if not impossible, to compare across studies.

A third limitation has to do with sources of information. Most studies use a parent or teacher as the informant (Kaffman & Elizur, 1983; Van Eerdewegh et al., 1982) but do not include responses from the children themselves. Although parents are reliable informants, their own grief may influence their observations. A further limitation has to do with sample sources. Most studies use small and unrepresentative samples of bereaved children (Felner et al., 1981; Kaffman & Elizur, 1983; Rutter, 1984) and study different age cohorts of children.

A final limitation has to do with research design. Although most of the studies listed above are prospective rather than retrospective, the majority are cross-sectional and not longitudinal (Kranzler et al., 1990). A longitudinal design is preferable because

1

children are growing and changing. In addition, bereavement, the adaptation to a loss, involves a process that takes place over time (Baker et al., 1992; Silverman, 1986). Any changes in the child's behavior relate not only to maturation but also to the time elapsed since the death (Silverman & Worden, 1992; Worden, 1991).

Dr. Phyllis Silverman, coprincipal investigator, and I designed the Child Bereavement Study to address limitations of previous studies in order to gain a clearer picture of the risk for seriously disturbed behavior in dependent school-age children losing a parent to death. The Child Bereavement Study is a prospective study of children between the ages of 6 and 17 who lost a parent to death. It involves a nonclinical representative community sample, interviewing both the surviving parent and all school-aged children in the family, following the family for 2 years after the death, and assessing a matched nonbereaved sample of children. We wanted to identify specific behaviors that are overrepresented in bereaved children when compared to controls, to determine whether these behaviors are possible consequences of parental loss, and to look at the implications of these behaviors for intervention.

THE PURPOSE OF THIS BOOK

In this book I want to present major findings from the Child Bereavement Study and to look at the implications of these findings for intervention with bereaved children and their families. Some of these findings support existing notions about bereaved children, whereas others do not. These contradictory findings point up the need for additional longitudinal studies of community-based samples of bereaved children, using nonbereaved controls, to bolster our understanding of the sequelae of parental death and the needs of bereaved children.

Part I, "Children and Their Families in Mourning," looks at findings from the Child Bereavement Study. Chapter 1 addresses the question "Do Children Mourn?" If so, at what age does this occur, and what does the process look like? What are the major influences on the course and outcome of childhood bereavement? Chapter 2 looks at the circumstances of the death, the families' rituals, and how these can influence the child's adjustment to the loss. Chapter 3 describes the families' experience of parental loss and how the changes brought about by this loss affected the children and their surviving parent during the first 2 years after the death. Chapter 4 looks at how the children themselves changed as they responded to the loss of a parent. The magnitude of the impact of loss is considered as the behavior of the bereaved children is compared with their nonbereaved counterparts. Chapter 5 outlines the important mediators of the bereavement experiences and looks at how these various mediators affected the course and outcome of bereavement. Chapter 6 explores to what extent experiencing parental death places children at risk for serious emotional and behavioral consequences. I also try to identify those parameters most likely to place children at risk. Risk profiles for bereaved children are outlined and a screening instrument is discussed to determine the children most at risk (see also Appendix B). In Part II, "Comparative Losses," children's reactions to the death of a parent are compared to the reactions of children experiencing other types of losses. In Chapter 7 children's loss of a sibling is compared with children's loss of a parent, while comparison of bereaved children and divorced children is made in Chapter 8. Part III addresses "How We Can Help Bereaved Children." Chapter 9 outlines the needs of grieving children that are the basis for grief counseling and looks at several issues that must be considered before such interventions may be undertaken. "Red-flag" behaviors that warrant further mental health evaluation for the child are also discussed. Chapter 10 looks at various models that can be used for intervention with bereaved children and their families, and at activities that will facilitate children through the various tasks of mourning. In the Epilogue we hear from the bereaved children regarding the counsel that they would give other children who are experiencing parental loss. In the end it is their wisdom, born of experience, that gives the best insight into children and grief.

THE CHILD BEREAVEMENT STUDY: METHODOLOGICAL OVERVIEW

Recruitment

Families were recruited from communities in the greater Boston area selected to represent a range of socioeconomic, religious, and ethnic backgrounds. During the recruiting period funeral directors in these communities invited to participate those families they served who met the criteria for inclusion in the study. These criteria included parents living together at the time of the death with children in the family between the ages of 6 and 17. We were able to identify, with few exceptions, every bereaved family in the selected target communities. Of those who received invitations to participate, 70 families (51%) accepted. There were no significant differences between the families who accepted and those who refused, based on gender and age of the deceased, suddenness of the death, family religion, and number of children. From a demographic point of view, the study population was a repre-sentative sample of bereaved families in these communities. We recognize, however, that factors other than demographic may influence the decision to participate. We must assume that there may be some bias in favor of people who see value in talking about their grief.

Assessment

Semistructured interviews with the children and their surviving parent were conducted in the family home at 4 months after the death and at the first and second anniversaries. Children were asked questions regarding their predeath status, experience with the death, mourning behavior, life changes since the death, school functioning, current health status, peer relationships, and attitudes of and behav-iors with other members of the family related to the loss. The parent interview covered family demography, predeath status, cir-cumstances of the death, mourning behavior, current support, an appraisal of stress and coping, concerns about the children, family activities, and responses to the death.

In addition to the interviews, standardized assessments of locus of control (Nowicki & Strickland, 1973), self-perception (Harter, 1979), and the child's understanding of death (Smilansky, 1987) were completed by the children. The surviving parent completed the following standardized instruments: Family Adaptability and Cohesion Evaluation Scales (FACES-III; Olson et al., 1985), meas-uring family cohesion and adaptability; Family Crisis Oriented Personal Evaluation Scales (F-COPES; McCubbin et al., 1987), measuring family coping; Family Inventory of Life Events (FILE; McCubbin et al., 1979), measuring family stressors and changes; Center for Epidemiological Studies—Depression Scale (CES-D; Radloff, 1977); Impact of Events Scale (IES; Zilberg et al., 1981); and, for each child, a Child Behavior Checklist (CBCL; Achenbach, 1991; Achenbach & Edelbrock, 1983). Details on these assessment instruments can be found in Appendix A.

Demography

We interviewed 70 families with 125 children among them between the ages of 6 and 17. Of these families, 50 experienced the death of a father and 20 the death of a mother. These figures are similar to national death statistics for the age cohort of these parents, where 2.5 men die for every 1 woman. There were an almost equal number of boys ($n = 65$) and girls ($n = 60$) in the sample who were attending the first through the twelfth grades; the average age of the children was 11.6 years. Of the children, 74% experienced father loss and 26% mother loss. At the time of death, 48% of the children were preteens and 52% were adolescents.

The average age of the surviving parent was 41 years, with a range of 30 to 57. For most of these couples (91%) this was their only marriage, and the length of marriage ranged from 2 to 36 years with a mean of 17 years. The number of children ranged from 1 to 5 with a mean of 2.5. There were nine children who had no siblings. The religious affiliation of this population reflected the large concentration of Roman Catholics in the greater Boston area. Of the families, 70% were Catholic, 23% Protestant, 6% Jewish, and 1% other.

From a socioeconomic point of view these families represented a cross-section of the communities studied. Family incomes after the death ranged from less than $10,000 a year to more than $50,000, with a modal income range of $20,000 to $29,000.

Deaths

Most of the deaths ($n = 62$) were from natural causes. There were five accidental deaths, two suicides, and one homicide. Of the deaths, 60% were expected and 40% were sudden. There were similar percentages of men and women in the sudden death category as in the expected death category. The proportion of men and women who had cared for a spouse during a long illness was also not significantly different. Of the 42 parents who died from a prolonged illness, 43% had been ill for over a year.

Nonbereaved Control Children

One major weakness of existing studies has been the lack of appropriate controls. To strengthen our study we were able to obtain a group of nonbereaved children that were matched with the bereaved children by age, gender, grade in school, family religion, and community. Control children were identified by school personnel from schools in the study communities and asked to participate in the investigation. We randomly selected one child from each of the 70 bereaved families and selected a matched control for that particular child. There were 70 control children in the study.

Attrition

Attrition was minimal over the 2-year follow-up period, with only four families and seven children leaving the study. This is a very low figure when compared to other longitudinal studies of bereavement and other longitudinal studies in general.

CHILDREN AND THEIR FAMILIES IN MOURNING

The Mourning Process
for Children

The death of a parent is one of the most fundamental losses a child can face. Ideally, parents support their children, both physically and emotionally; they provide a stable home environment in which children can grow and mature; and they serve both as the children's protectors and as their models. In reality, the extent to which parents fulfill these roles varies. Nevertheless, for the great majority of children, parents remain their most significant others; in effect, their partners in negotiating the essential developmental tasks that will take them to adulthood. The loss of a parent to death and its consequences in the home and in the family change the very core of the child's existence.

DO CHILDREN MOURN?

Most professionals agree that the ability to grieve is acquired in childhood as ego functions mature and the child is able to comprehend the finality of death. But there has been a lengthy and often contradictory debate among professionals as to when children acquire this capacity. On one side, people such as Wolfenstein (1966) believe that the capacity to mourn is not acquired until adolescence when the person is fully differentiated. On the other side of the debate, Bowlby (1963, 1980) posits that infants as young as 6 months experience grief reactions resembling those seen in adults. A middle position, represented by R. Furman (1964), places the capacity to mourn at around 3½ to 4 years of age.

9

Deutsch (1937), in her classic paper on the absence of grief, identified adults who had lost a parent in childhood and who reported a lack of appropriate emotions at the time of the loss. From her limited number of observations, she concluded that "the phenomenon of indifference is due to the fact that the ego of the child is not sufficiently developed to bear the strain of the work of mourning and it therefore utilizes some mechanism of narcissistic self-protection to circumvent the process" (pp. 227–228).

Part of the controversy focuses around the definition of mourning, which has been used with varying meanings in the literature of parental death. For example, psychoanalysts such as Wolfenstein (1966) posit that mourning involves the task of detaching from the attachment object and recognizing oneself as a separate entity. Likewise, Anna Freud (1960) subscribes to a highly specialized meaning of the term that involves withdrawal of libido from the lost object. For both analysts, young children cannot mourn because they have limited ego capacities such as reality testing, and lack of control of id tendencies. However, unlike the position usually taken by the psychoanalytic schools, some theorists, such as Kliman (1968), do not see mourning in terms of outcome, but rather as a broad spectrum of responses set into motion with the death of a loved one. Despite differences, however, most would agree that the child must have achieved a coherent mental representation of important attachment figures, such as parents, as well as object constancy for mourning to occur. Most children develop these capacities by 3 or 4 years of age.

MOURNING AND THE CHILD'S UNDERSTANDING OF DEATH

The child's comprehension of death and the role this comprehension plays in the process of mourning is a major component in our understanding of childhood bereavement. Concepts such as finality, causality, and irreversibility are abstractions, the understanding of which is clearly related to a child's cognitive development (E. Furman, 1974; Piaget, 1954; Smilansky, 1987).

In her classic study on the subject, Nagy (1948, 1959) posits three distinct conceptual stages of childhood mourning: Stage 1 (ages 3 to 5) when the child sees death as departure with the deceased existing somewhere else, Stage 2 (ages 5 to 9) when death is personified and can sometimes be avoided, and Stage 3 (ages 9 or 10) when the child understands that death is inevitable and affects all people, including him- or herself.

More recent researchers hold that certain children develop a realistic understanding of death much earlier than Nagy suggested. For example, Spinetta and Deasey-Spinetta (1981) and Bluebond-Langner (1978), who work with seriously ill children, note mature understandings of death in children between 6 and 10 years of age.

Researchers such as R. Furman, who believe that very young children can grieve, emphasize other factors that facilitate such mourning: It is more likely to occur in an environment where family members, particularly a consistent adult, reliably satisfy the child's reality needs and encourage the expression of sad affect. Some go as far as to say that it is not necessary for a child to have a realistic concept of death in order to grieve. Schell and Loder-McGough state that the focus should be placed on separation and the emotional response to separation. Such reactions can be seen quite apart from the cognitive development of the child.

In the Child Bereavement Study we took the position that a certain process begins when a child loses a parent to death. We wanted to look at this process both as described by children themselves and as described by their surviving parent. It was our hope that with a more thorough understanding of the process it would be possible to identify the specific interventions that may facilitate the adaptation of bereaved children to their loss.

In this book (and in the Boston study) I define "bereavement" as the adaptation to the loss, and "mourning" as the process children go through on their way to adaptation. I use the term "grief" to describe the child's personal experience, thoughts, and feelings associated with the death. Although similarities were found among children's experience, there was, as one would expect, a wide range of grief experiences.

TASKS OF MOURNING FOR CHILDREN

If mourning is defined as the process of adaptation to loss, what does this process look like in children? Readers who are familiar with my earlier book, *Grief Counseling and Grief Therapy* (Worden, 1982, 1991), will recognize the concept of the "tasks of mourning." Borrowing from developmental psychology, I conceive of the mourning process as consisting of four tasks. The bereaved must grapple with and bring some degree of resolution to each of these tasks as part of their overall adaptation to loss. Tasks do not have to be accomplished in any specific order and they can be revisited and reworked by the grieving person over time. The use of a task model is superior to a stage or phase model because of its dynamic fluidity and because it is a useful model for the clinician who may be intervening with bereaved individuals and families.

Do tasks of mourning apply to bereaved children? My answer would be a qualified "Yes"—they do apply but they can only be understood in terms of the cognitive, emotional, and social development of the child. Loss through death is experienced and expressed in different ways at different developmental phases. For example, a child who has not developed the cognitive abstractions of irreversibility and finality will have difficulty with Task I, accepting the reality of the loss. When dealing with the emotional impact of the loss (Task II), a child age 4 or 5 with magical thinking may believe that he or she caused the death to happen and must deal with guilt from this belief. This is less likely to happen once the child moves beyond the magical thinking stage. A young child with less well-developed coping skills may take longer than an older child to adjust to an environment where the deceased is missing (Task III). Children renegotiate the relationship with their dead parent over time, as they pass through the various developmental mileposts in their lives (Silverman, 1989), and this affects the way they deal with Task IV, emotionally relocating the deceased.

Researchers who apply my "tasks of mourning" concept to children have suggested various numbers of mourning tasks. Fox (1985) identified five tasks of mourning whereas Wolfelt (1996) and Baker et al. (1992) identified six. Although their conceptualizations are interesting, I do not believe we need to include additional tasks. The issues concerning bereaved children can be subsumed under the four tasks of mourning described in my earlier work, but I have modified them here to take into account the age and developmental level of the child.

Task I: To Accept the Reality of the Loss

When there is a death, adults often experience disbelief that the death has occurred. This is heightened in the case of a sudden death or a death in which no body is retrieved, or when the survivor does not see the loved person dead. The sense of disbelief can range from a hope that the loss hasn't occurred to a full delusion that the person is not dead at all. It is not unusual to hear a car pull into the driveway and to think it is the loved one, only to have to remind oneself that the person is dead. An adult whose parent has died may want to share some experience with the deceased and reach for the telephone, only to realize that they can no longer simply pick up the phone and talk to the parent. Over time, however, adults come to realize and accept that their lost loved one is dead and is not coming back.

Like adults, children must believe that the deceased is indeed dead and will not return to life before they can deal with the emotional impact of a loss. "I always forget and I think he's going to come through the door or something but he doesn't. It's, like, hope and then it's just, like, rejection again." This requires that the child comprehend the nature of abstractions such as finality and irreversibility, an understanding that only emerges when the child is capable of operational thinking (Piaget, 1954). An awareness of one's relationship to the physical and social world is acquired through reality testing, and young children who do not yet have this capacity may also have difficulty understanding the reality of the loss. For example, they may believe that the parent is just "away" and will return, as if from a business trip or a vacation.

To negotiate the first task of mourning, children need to be told about the death in ways that are accurate and in language that is age appropriate. They also need to be told repeatedly over time. The repetitive questions that children often ask about a death are a way for them to grapple with the reality of the death, as well as a test to be sure that the story has not changed. Children who are not given accurate information make up a story to fill in the gaps. Sometimes this can be more extreme and more frightening to the child than what actually happened.

As children develop cognitively, they acquire the ability to understand the finality of loss. "I thought when she died, 'It's all a dream,' and then I wake up and it's true," said a 10-year-old boy who lost his mother. But with both children and adults, there is always the delicate balance between wishing that it had not happened, or that the deceased will return, and the reality of the loss.

Task II: To Experience the Pain or Emotional Aspects of the Loss

It is necessary to acknowledge and work through the variety of emotions associated with the loss or these affects will manifest in other ways, perhaps somatically or in aberrant behavior patterns. Children need to approach this task gradually and in ways that do not overwhelm their coping capacity, which is generally less well developed than that of adults. Children between the ages of 5 and 7 years are a particularly vulnerable group. Their cognitive development enables them to understand something of the permanency of death, but they still lack the ego and social skills to deal with the intensity of the feelings of loss. One 6-year-old girl began having nightmares and high levels of anxiety after she learned her mother had less than 6 months to live. Her 3-year-old brother and 13-year-old sister did not experience such anxiety. Although she was sent to Sunday school in order to have a better understanding of what death is, her high levels of anxiety continued long after the mother's death.

Affects experienced by children are similar to those of adults. They may express sadness, anger, guilt, anxiety, and other feelings associated with loss. A child's ability to process the pain of loss will be influenced by observing the adult's experience of this process. If the child sees an adult express grief without being overwhelmed, this can serve as a salutary model for the child. On the other hand, if children see adults dysfunctional with grief, they may be frightened of feelings in general and their own feelings in particular.

Counselors who work with bereaved children should also pay particular attention to feelings of ambivalence and responsibility. If a highly ambivalent relationship existed between the child and the deceased parent prior to the death, one often finds considerable anger, frequently expressed in feelings of abandonment such as "Why did he [or she] leave me?" Ambivalent relationships may also lead children to feel responsible for the death because of something they did or did not do or say. Identifying such feelings and helping the child to reality test them is an important task of the bereavement counselor.

Task III: To Adjust to an Environment in Which the Deceased Is Missing

The nature of this adjustment is determined by the roles and relationships that the dead parent played in the child's life, as well as in the life of the family. For example, the mother is frequently the emotional caretaker of the family as well as the child's confidante. An aspect of the mourning process includes adapting to the loss of these roles, which have died with the mother. For most children, including those in the Boston study, the death of a mother results in more daily life changes than the death of a father. These changes significantly affect the child's emotional outlook and create major disruptions to which the child must adjust.

For children, this adjustment goes on over time. As they mature into adolescence, they realize in new ways what has been lost to parental death (Silverman, 1989). Mourning for a childhood loss can be revived at many points in life, especially when important life events reactivate the loss. For example, a girl whose father dies when she is 9 years old may realize anew what this loss means when she prepares to marry at age 23 and she must adjust to a situation in which her father is not there to participate in the wedding. Other realizations arise when she has her first child or goes through other transitional points of adulthood.

Task IV: To Relocate the Dead Person within One's Life and Find Ways to Memorialize the Person

The widely accepted notion that the bereaved need to "let go" of the deceased confuses our understanding of the mourning process. Freud wrote that the function of mourning is to "detach the survivor's hopes and memories from the dead" (1917, p. 65), and while this may be partially true, it is also true that one never forgets a significant relationship. The task facing the bereaved is not to give up the relationship with the deceased, but to find a new and appropriate place for the dead in their emotional lives—one that enables them to go on living effectively in the world (Marris, 1974; Shuchter & Zisook, 1986; Worden, 1991).

Children seek not only an understanding of the meaning of death but also a sense of who this now–dead parent is in their lives. While the loss of a parent is permanent and unchanging, the process is not; it is part of the child's ongoing experience (Silverman et al., 1992). The child must be helped to transform the connection to the dead parent and to place the relationship in a new perspective, rather than to separate from the deceased. "Does everyone die? Yes, physically, but not in your heart. If you admire the person that much you can say, 'No, they are not dead [in my heart]; only a 'wacko' person would feel that way and I don't feel that way about Mom," said a teenage boy who was struggling with this fourth task of mourning.

MEDIATORS OF THE MOURNING PROCESS

Although I have delineated four major tasks of mourning, it is clear that each child will negotiate these tasks in his or her own individual way. There is a wide range of normal responses to the death of a parent, and the personal circumstances of each child will influence the way in which he or she ultimately deals with the loss. Most, but not all, children manage the tasks of mourning in a healthy fashion. However, during the first 2 years after the death, a significant minority of children in the Child Bereavement Study (33%) was found to be at some degree of risk for high levels of emotional and behavioral problems.

Different children have different sources of support and strength, and different areas of vulnerability. Adjustment to loss is multidetermined. Although these determinants interact in complex and subtle ways, it is possible to identify six major categories of mediators that influence the course and outcome of adaptation to loss. These mediators are as follows:

1. The death and the rituals surrounding it
2. The relationship of the child with the deceased parent both before the death and afterward
3. The functioning of the surviving parent and his or her ability to parent the child

4. Family influences such as size, solvency, structure, style of coping, support, and communication, as well as family stressors and changes and disruptions in the child's daily life
5. Support from peers and others outside the family
6. Characteristics of the child including age, gender, self-perception, and understanding of death

Variations in these mediating factors mean variations in the mourning process for each individual child and will determine the way a child experiences grief following the loss of a parent. In the following chapters I will discuss how these influences played out in the lives of the children in the Child Bereavement Study. Chapters 5 and 6 take a close look at the most important mediators that have clinical utility in predicting a child's experience.

POINTS TO REMEMBER:
THE MOURNING PROCESS FOR CHILDREN

• The ability to mourn is acquired in childhood as ego functions mature and the child is able to comprehend the finality of death.

• There are different opinions as to when children develop the capacity to grieve, but many now think that children mourn earlier than was once believed.

• A key component in children's grief is their emotional reaction to separation. This exists very early and may predate a realistic concept of death.

• Childhood grief is best facilitated in the presence of a consistent adult who is able to meet the child's needs and to help the child express feelings about the loss.

• The mourning process in children involves four tasks of mourning that are influenced by the developmental issues of the growing child.

• Children's reactions to the death of a parent can vary in terms of intensity and duration. Six major categories of mediating factors contribute to the specific grief reactions of a given child.

T · W · O

When a Parent Dies

When a parent dies, life as the child knows it is disrupted and irrevocably changed. This is likely to be a time of pain and confusion, both for children and the surviving parent. "I came home from school to find the house full of people. My uncle told me my father had died suddenly. I was so shocked and confused, I went upstairs and worked on my geometry," said one teenage boy.

Although most children need to face common hurdles, such as learning of the death and attending the funeral, each child's experience of the time following the death will be shaped by a broad range of mediating factors. Among these are the specific circumstances of the death and the way in which the surviving family members cope with the crisis. In this chapter I will discuss these as well as the child's relationship with the dead parent after the loss. Each of these mediators can have a significant impact on the adaptation to the loss.

LEARNING OF THE DEATH

Children vary in their emotional and behavioral reactions at the time of loss, but their responses are strongly influenced by those of the surviving parent and other adults. Learning of the death is a significant moment in the bereavement process. Three-quarters of the children in the Child Bereavement Study were told of the death by their surviving parent. "When Mother called me to tell me

18

Dad died, I told her she was a liar. I was frightened. I started shaking," said a 9-year-old girl. Others were informed in various ways, usually by another family member. The study included 15 children who were present when their parent died.

On hearing of the death, children in the Boston study were varied in their emotional responses. When the death occurred without warning, they described their reactions with words such as "shocked," "stunned," or "I just couldn't believe it." One teen, who was told of the death by a cousin, thought it was a cruel joke and seemed confused as to how to react. "I just thought it couldn't be but went to school that day to sort of get my mind off it," reported a 14-year-old boy whose father died suddenly.

Most children, both boys and girls, cried when they heard the news. "I felt sad that the praying didn't work. I went downstairs and cried for 20 minutes," said a 14-year-old boy. The rest of the children expressed their sadness through tears within a few days or weeks. "I didn't cry then. I cried 3 weeks later alone in my room," said a 9-year-old girl. Many children spoke of feeling sad and confused, even when the death was expected; others spoke of not knowing just how to respond. "Even though I was present when he died, I couldn't believe it." Some children expressed anger. On hearing that her father was dead, a 15-year-old girl reported, "I wasn't just mad. I was nasty." "I was angry that my mother took the pills and surprised that my father turned off the machine. I am still angry at her," an 11-year-old boy told us.

People choose different ways to deal with their feelings, and the children in this study were no exception. Some turned to their families, while others derived comfort from their friends. Some children withdrew and needed to be alone, either retreating to their rooms or going for a walk or a bicycle ride. "When I heard, I ran under my bunk bed and hid," stated an 8-year-old boy. "After hearing I cried. I went to my room by myself and thought things over. What am I going to do now? How can I help the family?" a teenage boy asked himself.

The reactions of the surviving parent had a great impact on the children's behavior. Many had never before seen their parent so upset and expressing such strong emotions. For some children this was very frightening. Many children (42%) felt the need to act in a certain way for the parent's benefit, and most followed through. Teenage boys, in particular, felt pressure to act strong for the surviving parent. "I felt like I had better act that it didn't affect me as much. It made her feel better. I don't think she wanted to see me as a total wreck," asserted a 16-year-old boy. Another teenage boy said, "For my father I tried not to cry as much. I tried to be good."

CIRCUMSTANCES OF THE DEATH

Whether the death is expected or sudden affects the family's responses to it. When there had been a long illness, children were less likely to cry on hearing the news, although they did cry later. Some expressed feelings of relief, especially when the parent had experienced considerable suffering.

Surviving parents were more likely than their children to be aware of the terminal nature of the illness and this affected the family in various ways. Women in the study were more likely to stop work when their husbands were very ill, and were also more likely to plan ahead, both financially and for the needs of the children. Most husbands with sick wives continued to work. In general, mothers seemed more in touch with the family's changing needs in the light of an impending death, and were more available to the children during this time.

Not all children were made aware of the terminal condition of the illness, and of those who were, most knew for a relatively brief time before the death. "I knew my father was ill but just didn't think that he would die," said a 13-year-old boy. Young children were least likely to know, while teenagers were most aware. When the parent died at home, children were more likely to know about the pending death for a longer period.

Most children who were told of the pending death were told by the nonsick parent. Some told the children directly: "Mother said, 'Dad's going to die. Don't tell him,' " reported a 6-year-old girl. Others were told in a more oblique manner, as was the teenage boy whose mother asked, "Would you mind going to the cemetery if someone you knew died?" He said, "I figured it out." Other children were told of the pending death by the sick parent.

"You know, there's going to come a time when I'm going to get really sick and I'm not going to be here anymore," a mother told her 15-year-old daughter. Another mother told her 12-year-old boy that she would die but she wanted them to go on living and do what they always did.

THE FUNERAL AND OTHER FAMILY RITUALS[1]

Family rituals are important mediators influencing the course and outcome of bereavement. A key family ritual is the funeral. The funeral can help meet three important needs of children around the time of a death. It provides (1) a means to acknowledge the death, (2) a way to honor the life of the deceased, and (3) a means of support and comfort for the bereaved children (Silverman & Worden, 1992). But children need to be prepared for the funeral if it is to be a positive part of the mourning process. They should be given a choice about whether to attend the viewing of the body, the funeral, and the burial, but need first to be clearly informed about what they will see and experience.

Acknowledging the Death

As outlined in Chapter 1, the first task of mourning is to acknowledge the reality of the loss. The funeral is a good place to begin this aspect of grief work. One teenage boy whose father died asserted, "It helped me realize that he was not coming back," and an 11-year-old boy said, "It was a way of sending her off to a better life." A 13-year-old girl, who had not been able to see her mother before the death, talked about the importance of seeing her at the viewing. Another teenage girl told of how the funeral helped her deal with the reality of her father's death: "I was glad I was there. People needed me, but I also went for myself. I needed to know what happened. This is it. Here is this hole. He is not alive anymore. I saw it."

[1]Parts of this section have previously appeared in Silverman and Worden (1992).

Honoring the Life of the Deceased

The funeral gives children the opportunity to honor their dead parent. Many children were aware of this when we interviewed them. A teenage boy said, "I'm his son. It would have been disrespectful not to be there." A boy who was 10 reiterated this thought: "He was my father and, no matter how young I was, I had to be there." There was a touching comment from a 6-year-old girl whose father killed himself: "If I wasn't at the funeral, he wouldn't know I loved him."

Providing Support

A funeral can provide support and comfort for the child. Many of the children were pleased that friends from school attended and felt that it was important that everyone participated and that they were able to mourn together: "The kids made cards for me and my teacher brought them in at the funeral place." Extended family members also provided support. One child reported, "At the end, while I was crying, my little cousin came up to me and gave me a hug and said it was okay. She was only 3." A teenage boy said, "The purpose is to get everyone feeling okay about it [the death]. Anybody who wanted to could come. It is for children too, a way for little kids to understand that people have a life on earth but they die." A teenage girl whose mother had died summed up this benefit of the funeral by saying, "Everyone gave me support. It made me feel better that all the people were there."

Participating in the Funeral

Some type of funeral or burial ritual was observed by nearly all of the families in the study. This is not surprising as families were recruited by funeral service personnel. Most Protestant families had a religious service either at the funeral home or at the church. The Catholic funerals included a mass at the church and a graveside service. Jewish funerals were traditional, with a closed casket, a service at the funeral home, and another at the graveside within 24 to 48 hours after the death. Buddhist families had a service in the home with the remains present as prescribed by their tradition.

A surprisingly large percentage (95%) of the children attended the funeral. In most families there was very little discussion about whether or not to include the children in this ritual. It was generally assumed that they would be there and they were. Children were included in funeral planning and in the funeral itself in various ways. This participation did not lead to later behavioral/emotional difficulties; on the contrary, most children felt positive about their involvement. Being included also helped children to feel important and useful at a time when many were feeling overwhelmed. A 10-year-old boy who helped carry his father's coffin said, "It was kinda heavy but it felt good to carry his coffin."

Some children were involved in making the funeral arrangements: "My son was 17. He helped me plan everything. We decided that when his father was in the casket if it didn't look like him, we would not open it. We agreed that he looked like himself and kept the casket open."

Other children selected the burial clothing or chose the flowers or music to be played at the service. One teenage girl helped pick out the casket and insisted on oak, because her craftsman father had enjoyed working with this type of wood. Children were less involved in decisions regarding burial or cremation, a decision that was made either by the deceased before the death or by the surviving parent.

Viewing of the body in an open casket was part of the religious and family tradition for many of these families. For most of the children the wake was the only time they were able to see the body of their dead parent. "It was scary at the wake 'cause it really didn't look like her," said a teenage girl. In order to make this a meaningful experience, some families arranged a private viewing for the children. This also gave the parent better control in case the children became too upset. Altogether, 78% of the children were able to view the deceased parent's body. Some children, like this 12-year-old boy, chose not to see their parent's body: "They said that I could go see my father dead at the hospital. I said, 'No,' because if I hugged him he couldn't hug back."

Of the six children who did not attend the funeral, four were under the age of 10, and the decision not to attend was made by the surviving parent. In these four cases of nonattendance the deaths had been sudden, and it is difficult to know whether the choices were based on the welfare of the children or on the surviving parent's difficulty with confronting what had happened.

Two of the six children were given the choice whether or not to attend and opted not to. One was a 12-year-old boy whose mother had committed suicide. He did not attend the service because he had been so upset seeing the mother's body at the viewing. Another was a 10-year-old boy who said, "I didn't go to the funeral after she died. I didn't want to see her or anything. That would put a lot of hurt in me."

Although most children attended the funeral, some parents felt that the actual burial would be too upsetting for them. Nine children who attended the funeral did not attend the burial service. Other children who were present at the cemetery chose to remain by the cars rather than participate in this final ritual. Those who did attend the burial reported that they were happy to be given the choice, and most reported being comfortable with this part of the ritual.

Children's Reflections on the Funeral

Shortly after the death, children's recollections of the funeral were generally vague, with most children unable to remember significant details. Younger children tended to remember specific, concrete things, such as the bed or box in which their parent lay, without being able to remember what it was called. They would know that a speech was given, but would have no recollection of what was said. They could remember that extended family members attended, and that people said, "I'm sorry," to them.

Older children gave more meaning to the event, but were still vague about the experience during the early months after the loss. One adolescent boy noted, "It was nice to see that so many people knew my father," while another child remembered her mother not being in pain any longer. On the whole, even older children gave very few details about the funeral and their involvement in it. It was difficult to discern whether these vague memories were a function of the general numbness that people experience around the time of death (Worden, 1991), or if they were due to the lack of preparation provided the children before the funeral, or simply to a reluctance to talk.

Recollections of the funeral had become clearer by the first anniversary of the death; and 2 years after the event, children could acknowledge and talk more easily about their feelings at the time. Nearly all the children who attended (95%) felt good about what had gone on at the funeral.

As a way to get the children to think about the funeral and to evaluate it from their own perspective, we asked them 2 years after the death if they would, in retrospect, redesign or modify their parent's funeral in some way. Half of the children gave us a redesigned funeral. Those who did were more likely to show little or no disturbed behavior on the CBCL during the 2-year period. They also came from families in which the surviving parent had experienced lower levels of stress and depression during the same bereavement period.

What were the changes that children wanted in the funeral? Many wanted it to be more of a reflection of the parent who died. A young girl whose father was an environmentalist was disappointed that nothing in the service reflected his passion. She redesigned the funeral to be in the mountains to show this side of her father. Some children wanted the funeral to be larger with more people who could honor the life of their parent. They were aware of the number of people attending the service and found comfort in knowing that their parent was well liked. One teenage girl said, "A funeral is like a rock concert. If no one comes, it's not a good concert." A girl who was 8 when her father died confided, "So many people came. My dad had a lot of friends." However, other children believed that a smaller funeral was the best way to honor the parent, an intimate service that included only immediate family members.

Some children wanted to change the somber, dark, and downbeat atmosphere of the funeral. One child wanted the funeral to have bright colors to help people remember the good things. Another child redesigned the funeral to be on the beach surrounded by exquisite flowers. "Mother loved the beach. There everybody would pay respect and show they loved her. It would be good to be on the beach—not so boring."

The viewing was unpleasant for some of the children and they wanted to change it. "I wouldn't have the casket open; he was all pale and everything," a 9-year-old girl said. Children in another family were upset by the way the mother looked at the wake. She hadn't worn much makeup in life and was wearing bright crimson lipstick in the casket.

More than two-thirds of the children had revisited the grave in the early months after the death, and this number increased significantly (85%) by the end of the first year of bereavement. Some passed the cemetery on the way home from school and would stop to visit. "I usually went there when I felt sad and when I needed someone to talk to," reported a 12-year-old girl whose father died. Others went not for themselves but to help other family members. "I don't like going to the cemetery, but I go just for my mother. Because that's just where his body is. It's not him," said a 13-year-old girl. Those who visited were more likely to come from families who spoke easily about the deceased, who commemorated the first anniversary of the death, and who included the children in the planning of this commemoration.

There was a slight decline (78%) in cemetery visits during the second year of bereavement. Children most likely to be visiting at this point were those who had lost a mother and those who reported a closer relationship with their surviving parent. One teenage boy who had never been to the grave during this 2-year period held this option in reserve: "If I was, like, really depressed and I need to see it and I need to talk to him, I would go."

There were 10 families who did not use earth burial but cremated the deceased and disposed of the ashes in various ways. In one family the father's ashes were scattered in the ocean. His 14-year-old son thought this was a good idea: "We went to the beach [where Father's ashes were scattered earlier]. It's like, wow, that's pretty neat. There's someone out there . . . he's all over the place."

THE ONGOING RELATIONSHIP
TO THE DEAD PARENT[2]

One of the tasks of mourning—Task IV—is not to give up the relationship with the deceased but to find a new and appropriate place for the dead in one's emotional life (Worden, 1991). The

[2]Parts of this section have previously appeared in Silverman et al. (1992).

Child Bereavement Study has extended our knowledge of the way in which children maintain an ongoing connection to the dead parent. Through a process we call "constructing" the deceased, the child develops an inner representation of the dead parent that allows him or her to maintain a relationship with the deceased, a relationship that changes as the child matures and the intensity of grief lessens. The child negotiates and renegotiates the meaning of the loss, and in time, relocates the dead person in his or her life and memorializes that person in a way that allows life to move on (Worden, 1991).

The following five dimensions of connection to the dead parent were identified and reported by Silverman et al. (1992):

1. Making an effort to locate the deceased
2. Experiencing the deceased
3. Reaching out for a connection
4. Remembering the deceased
5. Attaching to the deceased through transitional objects

Locating the Deceased

When asked where the dead parent was presently, most of the children in the study (74%), regardless of religious orientation, were able to locate the deceased, often "in heaven." Adolescents were less inclined to believe their parent was in a specific place, with adolescent girls being most skeptical of this notion in the early months after the death. In the 2 years following the death there was a shift in the perception of where the dead parent was located, with an increase in skepticism on the part of certain children. This shift may be related to developmental changes and growth, particularly as more children had become adolescents and teens continued to be the most skeptical group. A large number of children (68%), however, continued to believe that their parent resided in a specific place.

There was considerable speculation about the nature of this specific place. A 10-year-old boy whose mother died pondered, "I want to know what it is like up there. I think it must be peaceful and very quiet." An 11-year-old girl told us, "At night I think about what heaven would be like. Would it be like fields and

flowers, or would it be different for each family so you could see
all your other relatives?" Some children saw heaven as an extension
of life on earth. "If there are beaches in heaven, she's lying on a
beach somewhere, or maybe in an arts and crafts shop," said a
teenage girl of her mother. Others were content to find heaven
imponderable, as was one teenage boy who asserted, "Heaven is
like the Bermuda Triangle. We can't understand that."

Experiencing the Deceased

Feeling watched by the dead parent was a common experience,
particularly in the early months after the death. Those continuing
to feel watched 1 and 2 years after the death were more likely to
have lost mothers.

Many of the children who felt watched shortly after the loss
found this experience scary. Much of this fear had to do with the
belief that the dead parent would not approve of what they were
doing. One 11-year-old boy said, "I sometimes think that he is
watching me and it scares me because he might see me do
something he wouldn't like. . . . If someone's watching you, you
don't do it if it's bad." A teenage girl thought that her mother
would yell at her from heaven if she did not do well in school.
Some children interpreted sights and sounds happening around
them as indications of the presence of the dead parent.

For a few children the "presence" had more the flavor of being
haunted by the dead parent. "When I am alone in the house, I
get scared. The cellar has been turned into my room and there's a
little tiny room where we put stuff. I feel like she's always right
there behind the door waiting for me to come in." Similar feelings
were expressed by an 11-year-old boy: "When I wake up early in
the morning and it's really quiet, I always think that she is in the
room. Like, I get really scared like she's waking up from the dead.
I try to get dressed as fast as I can so I can run downstairs because
there are people down there." The same child said, "When I look
in the mirror in the morning to comb my hair, I always think that
she is going to pop up and scare me." A teenage boy admitted, "I
am scared of spirits. I sleep with the radio on and a baseball bat."
Over time the experience of being watched by the dead parent
became less frightening for these children.

It is interesting to note that many children endowed their dead parent with attributes associated with the living, such as hearing, seeing, feeling, and moving. A 14-year-old Catholic boy said, "I want my father to see me perform my magic shows. If I said a dead person can't see, then I would not be able to have my wish that he see what I am doing. I believe that the dead see, hear, move. Don't ask me how, I just believe it." A 17-year-old Jewish girl agreed, "Yes, the dead can see and hear. It's what I would like to think so my father could hear comforting words and maybe he can see significant events in my life."

Dreaming is another way children experienced the deceased. Over half the children in the study dreamed of their parent during the 4 months after the death, and many of these same children were still dreaming about the parent 2 years later. For most, the parent appeared alive in the dream, but this did not always bring comfort: "I dreamed he met me on the way home from school and that he hugged me. When I woke up, I felt so sad that I won't have that anymore." Other children derived consolation from these dreams: "When I wake up from these dreams, I know she's gone; but when I dream, it feels like she is there and it is reality."

Children who maintained a connection with the parent through dreams and feeling watched knew, for the most part, that these experiences were coming from something inside themselves. Nevertheless, this "middle knowledge" (Weisman, 1972) provided an effective compromise between an unpleasant truth and a wished-for state of events.

Reaching Out to the Deceased

Some children (57%) maintained a connection to their deceased parent by speaking to them, although the number of these children dropped significantly (39%) after the first anniversary of the death.

The style of speaking to the dead parent varied. One teenage girl would speak to her mother every time she walked past her mother's picture in the house. A 10-year-old boy reported, "In my mind I talk to him. I tell him what I did today, about the fish I caught, and that I did real good." A 10-year-old girl said she says good night to her father every night.

For many children, the cemetery is the last earthly contact with their parent, and some children chose to go there to speak to the deceased. A 12-year-old girl whose mother died said, "I go to the cemetery when I feel sad and I need someone to talk to." A 15-year-old boy often stopped by the cemetery on his way home from school: "I don't talk about it much, but I stop by to visit about once a week. I tell my father about my day and the things that I've done." Another teenage boy stated, "I ask him for advice. I talk to him kinda like he is God. I ask him to make things better."

Some children believed that they received responses or information from the dead parent, but the content was often vague. For example, a 16-year-old girl said, "My mother was my friend. I could talk to her about anything. I talk to her but she can't respond. She doesn't tell me what to do but she helps me. I can't explain it exactly." A similar experience was reported by an 11-year-old girl, who said, "If I have a problem, I talk to her. I ask her how she is doing even though she can't answer me. But I hear a voice in my head and know that she's doing fine."

Remembering the Deceased

Remembering and reflecting on the deceased is common to most bereaved people. Four months after the loss, nearly all children in the study (90%) thought about their dead parent several times a week; and, despite some decline, the frequency of thoughts remained at a high level (65%) 2 years following the death. Many children reminisced about activities they enjoyed with that parent, such as going to a favorite restaurant every Saturday for lunch. In some ways this is an acknowledgment of the reality of the death (Task I), that the person is gone, and that they won't ever share this activity again. Some children thought it was important to think less about their dead parent as they passed through the bereavement process. "I don't constantly think about it because I'd be hiding in myself and never get on with life," said a boy who was 10 when his father died.

Attaching through Transitional Objects

Most children (77%) kept something that belonged to their parent. This might have been given to the child by the dead parent or by the surviving parent, or it might have been appropriated by the child. A 10-year-old boy took his father's Little League pin: "I wanted to remember him because he liked baseball." His 11-year-old sister took a country music tape: "We used to listen to it together." This same girl felt somewhat left out because her brothers got the father's "personal things." She, however, found her own special niche in the family, telling us, "I am the closest to Mom, since I am the only girl in the family." Another teenage girl took some of her father's shirts and wore them around the house most of the time. She was upset when her mother gave her father's clothes away: "She didn't ask me and I didn't like it." An 11-year-old girl said, "I have a little stuffed rabbit that was given to my mother. She kept it in her room so I just went in and took it one day. I keep it in my room."

For the most part, these objects were kept close at hand during the early months after the loss. As the first year of mourning progressed, they became less important and took on the characteristics of keepsakes (Worden, 1991). A boy who wore his father's baseball cap at all times, including sleeping, when we interviewed him at 4 months was not wearing his father's cap at 1 year, but had it hanging on the bed post. At 2 years the cap resided in the closet.

Volkan (1981) used the term "linking objects" to refer to objects that keep the mourner living in the past. However, one might find a more positive meaning in the term "transitional objects"; these are seen as connecting one realm of experience with another (Winnicott, 1953; Worden, 1991). This was closer to the experience of these children.

Highly Connected Children

Some children were more connected to their dead parent than others. In the Child Bereavement Study we found that children who lost a parent of the same gender were more likely to stay connected to that parent. The most attached children were those who lost mothers rather than fathers, and were more likely to be girls than boys. Overall, adolescent boys were the least likely to stay connected.

Children who were highly connected at 4 months after the death continued to be so 2 years later. Highly connected children were better able to show their emotional pain, to talk with others about the death, and to accept support from families and friends. They were also more likely to visit the gravesite and to observe anniversaries of the death, and to try to please the dead parent with their behavior. When asked which of their parents they were most like, these children were more likely to select the deceased and frequently reported that they shared interests with this parent. "I look like my father so I do the same stuff as he did," said a 10-year-old boy who had enjoyed fishing with his father and kept his father's rod and tackle. "People remember him by looking at me." However, highly connected children also reported more uneasiness about the safety of their surviving parent and more sadness and crying. Although connection with the deceased is comforting, it does not preclude the experiencing of painful affect, nor does it result in fewer emotional/behavioral problems.

Constructing a connection to the deceased is a process that involves family members talking about the loss. Highly connected children tended to come from families that were rated closer and more cohesive. These families experienced lower levels of stress and there was an emphasis on religious and spiritual support. In such families both the surviving parent and the child were willing to talk about, to memorialize, and to relocate the lost member as part of the family process. One particularly moving vignette happened in the life of a 10-year-old boy who had difficulty talking about his dead father with other family members. His mother helped him to develop a positive memory of his father: "She says we'll pray every night for Daddy and that he'll be able to see me. She says we have to remember Daddy outside in the sunshine laughing, not like he looked when he died. I asked if Daddy can help me now, if he'll always be with me. Mom said, 'Yes.'"

POINTS TO REMEMBER:
WHEN A PARENT DIES

• The emotional responses and behaviors of children are varied around the time of loss but are strongly influenced by the reactions of the surviving parent and other adults.

- When a parent is in a terminal condition, the least likely to know are the younger children, and children are less likely to know than are the adults.
- Recapturing memories of the funeral and being able to talk about it increases over time for most children.
- Most children participated in the funeral ritual, and this participation did not lead to later emotional/behavioral difficulties. Those who were prepared for the funeral had fewer overall emotional and behavioral problems.
- Sudden and violent deaths are more likely to lead to indecision about funeral attendance by parents and children.
- Children who redesigned the funeral wanted the funeral to reflect the life of the individual more rather than to focus on the loss itself or the afterlife.
- Including children in the planning of the funeral has a positive effect, helping them to feel important and useful at a time when many are feeling overwhelmed.
- Children should be given a choice as to attending the wake, funeral, and burial; but these need to be informed choices, with children prepared for what they will see and experience.
- Visiting the grave can be an avenue for children to remain connected with the dead parent during a time when they are working through the place of the deceased in their current life.
- Children who remained connected after the loss are better able to talk about the dead parent both inside and outside the family, and are likely to try to please the dead parent with their behavior.
- An ongoing relationship with the deceased can be a healthy part of the process called "constructing."
- The constructing process involves renegotiating the meaning of the loss rather than "letting go" of the deceased; this renegotiation continues to be part of the child's life experience.
- Most children locate the deceased in a specific place such as "heaven," and endow the deceased with attributes of the living, although they make a distinction between body and soul.
- Children often feel "watched" by or have dreams about their deceased parent; most realize these are generated inside themselves.
- Communication with and memories of the deceased parent

are important in the mourning process and diminish over time, as does the significance of transitional objects.

• Children who are highly connected to the deceased parent seem better able to show their emotional pain, to talk with others about the death, and to accept support from family and friends. Although they experience emotional pain, this does not mean they are experiencing difficulty in the mourning process.

T·H·R·E·E

How Life Changes

When a parent dies, life changes for the child, the surviving parent, and the family. The child continues to live his or her everyday life within a family that is now missing a vital member. The family is an interactional unit in which all members influence each other, and the death of a parent has an impact on the entire family system. Most families exist in some type of homeostatic balance; and the loss of a significant person, together with the roles played by that person, can imbalance this system.

The child's adjustment to the death is inextricably intertwined with the way in which the family, and especially the surviving parent, responds to this loss. How does the surviving parent cope with becoming a single parent? In what ways does the child's relationship with the surviving parent affect the way in which the two together negotiate the reality of life without the deceased parent? Family members need to confront the death together so that the family as a whole can readjust as a working system after the loss.

THE CHALLENGE OF SINGLE PARENTING

With the death of a spouse, the surviving parent is thrust into a new role, that of single parent. At this very difficult period in their

Portions of this chapter have previously appeared in Worden and Silverman (1992).

lives, bereaved parents must deal not only with their own reactions to the death, but must respond to their child's needs as well. The degree to which a parent can meet both sets of needs will affect how well the child accommodates to the loss and to subsequent changes in his or her life.

Researchers have observed that bereaved children need three things to help them cope with the disruption in the family system caused by the death of a parent. These are (1) support (Brown et al., 1986; Elizur & Kaffman, 1983), (2) nurturance (Siegel et al., 1990), and (3) continuity (Reese, 1982). The child will feel supported when the parent can function as a teacher and guide, providing feedback and encouragement about the child's feelings and behavior following the death. A nurturing parent not only provides food, clothing, and shelter but is there to listen and use this information to help the child. Continuity is frequently overlooked when considering children's needs after a death. Though their world is forever changed, each bereaved child needs a sense that the family will continue, with a connection between the past and the future.

It is obvious that the surviving parent's ability to respond to a child's needs would be adversely affected by depression or some kind of mental or physical illness. Indeed, as discussed in Chapter 6, this puts a child at risk for poor adaptation to the loss. However, even normal grieving can limit the parent's responsiveness. Sadness, preoccupation with the deceased, and the pain associated with the loss all affect parents' ability to meet the needs of their children.

Men and women often respond to loss differently. Cook (1988) has noted that men who had lost a child were more solitary in their grief work and less comfortable expressing their feelings about the death. Generalizing from these findings, one would expect that mothers and fathers who survive the death of a spouse might face that death differently, and that the levels of openness in their respective families would reflect this difference.

The ways in which men and women respond to loss of a spouse are bound up with the different meanings the loss of the marital relationship has for bereaved men and women (Silverman, 1986). Women's sense of self is more likely to be framed by this relationship, but, at the same time, women are used to being the keepers of the family's emotional life. Men have a more difficult time living alone and handling daily household routines. As expected, men in the Boston study were more reticent about sharing their feelings. This clearly had implications for the child who was also negotiating the loss.

Physical Availability

A key determinant of whether bereaved children receive sufficient support is the physical availability of the surviving parent. Most families depend on the father as their primary means of economic support. Although some men in the study reduced their work hours during the final weeks before the death of their spouse, most did not stop working and resumed or continued full-time work after the death.

By contrast, the surviving mothers were likely to leave work entirely or change to part-time employment in order to be more available to their children after the death of the father. Women were also more likely to quit work to be at home during their spouse's illness. Although financial security was an issue for these families, we found that women in this study were more likely than men to have additional income from life insurance and social security. Mothers who worked outside the home were clear that they needed flexible hours so that they could be at home at the same times as their children. One mother said, "I had flexible hours. If anyone was sick or needed me after school, I was able to be there. I needed to work enough hours to get health insurance." Those mothers who continued to work full time also emphasized the need for flexibility. A few worked in the school system and had the same schedules as their children.

Both men and women acknowledged that work provided them with a place where they could temporarily lose themselves. One father of teenage children who was eager to return to work admitted, "My escape was in going to work. I increased my hours to keep busy and to make up for the lost hours during the last weeks of her life. I didn't even think of the kids. It took me 6 months before I was aware that they had needs too."

Men and women who worked full time experienced tension between their children's need for them and the demands of the job. Most men felt that they could not afford to stop work. A father of two young children said, "I was worried and changed jobs to be closer to home. I wasn't sure how I would manage children and job . . . but I had no choice."

Fathers were the least prepared for the role of single parent. For most of them, being responsible for the care of their children was a new experience. These fathers tended to send the children back to school almost immediately after the funeral while they returned to work. Although this was related to the father's need to get back to his normal routine and to show that life continues in spite of the loss, it was also related to his not knowing what else to do with the children at this time. There were some exceptions, however. One father, who had always done the cooking and shopping while his wife was busy with volunteer work, saw his current domestic role as a continuation of the one he had had before she got sick.

Emotional Availability

In the Child Bereavement Study we found that mothers tended to be more sensitive to their children's needs than were fathers. In fact, even depressed women were likely to be more aware of their children's needs than nondepressed men. One father said, "I had no idea about getting children off to school or that I should be involved in this activity. It took me almost a year before I realized that they lost *their* mother. It wasn't only that I lost my wife."

Most men felt directly responsible for what would happen to their children: "I worry about my son getting his grades back up"; "I think about the babysitter and how to keep the house covered while I work . . . about getting everything done." However, they rarely talked about helping children with their feelings. The children themselves frequently found it difficult to approach their fathers about their feelings or dreams.

As we expected, parents who were depressed or preoccupied with their own feelings about the loss were less available to their children. This group constituted a significant proportion of the parents in the study. At 4 months after the death over half (56%) of the surviving parents were assessed as depressed on a standardized instrument (CES-D). This number dropped to 40% by the second anniversary of the death. Although depression levels were similar between men and women 4 months after the death, more women remained depressed at the first anniversary of the loss. Those with high depression scores had significantly lower incomes and found these incomes inadequate. They also had more younger children. There were no significant gender differences in depression levels by the second year.

Depressed parents were less able to share their feelings with others. They saw themselves as being under extreme stress and found that their coping efforts were not satisfactory. They worried about their ability to care for the children and to meet their needs. One depressed mother fretted, "I'm always afraid that there is not enough of me to go around. Sometimes they talk to me and I don't even hear." Women who were not depressed worried about the children as well: "Bringing up the kids on my own, I guess . . . makes you a mess. I'm wrecked. I worry about the kids emotionally . . . and I think the realization that he won't be coming back is fierce."

Parents felt more than just sadness; they felt the absence of their spouse as well. Another depressed mother said, "I have boys, and they need a father. My husband could moderate between them when they fought. Can I do that?" A father was clear about his deficiencies: "My boy was very close to his mother. I don't know if I can have that kind of relationship with him. I don't see myself taking care of him that way . . . but I am all he has."

However, as time passed, many parents who seemed depressed shortly after the death slowly became more aware of their children's needs. Men who had sought an outlet in their work told us how their children finally reminded them that they were needed at home. One father, who earlier had not been able to articulate his feelings, said, "I try to be home for supper every night. I told my oldest boy he was not his kid brother's father, that was my job and I was here to do it. My wife overprotected our youngest. I'm letting him take his bike out of the driveway, and he's learning to visit friends by himself. He's 11 years old and he has to learn to do something on his own." Yet another father was pleased with all he had learned: They were getting meals on the table, the house was kept in some order, kids were getting off to school, and his oldest was starting college.

THE CHILD'S RELATIONSHIP
WITH THE SURVIVING PARENT

The death of a parent significantly affects a child's relationship with the remaining parent. Clearly, the physical and emotional availability of the surviving parent has a great influence on the child's relationship with that parent. The Child Bereavement Study showed that the gender of the surviving parent and the ages of the children are key factors in the dynamics of this changing relationship. In some families this relationship becomes closer, while in others the surviving parent becomes the target for the child's anger and acting-out behavior. We found both types of relationships in the study.

At 1 year after the death, two-thirds of the children reported that they felt closer to the surviving parent than to any other family member. Those reporting this closeness, not surprisingly, were more likely to be younger children, particularly preteen girls. Older children, especially adolescent boys, reported the least closeness to the surviving parent. In general, adolescents were more likely to select a sibling over a parent as their closest family member.

When asked to identify the parent to whom they were closest *before* the death, half of the children would not commit to an answer or said they were equally close to both of their parents. Of those who did make a selection, children who had experienced mother loss were twice as likely to select the dead parent over the surviving parent, while those who lost a father were equally distributed between the two choices. Overall, 61% of those bereaved children who made a selection reported that they felt closer to the deceased parent prior to the death than they felt to the surviving parent.

Many children, and adolescent boys in particular, observed that their surviving parent had changed during the first year of bereavement. A strong correlate of this observed change was an increase in tension with that parent. "My father used to be wicked nice and now he's, like, grouchy all the time," said a 12-year-old girl. "My sister moved out. She tried hard to act like a substitute mother but it didn't work out. She tried too hard." "Mother gets mad a lot and I try to make her happy," said a 6-year-old boy. A 14-year-old girl told us, "My mom seems more irritable and impatient. She starts crying and goes into her room. It makes me upset like I had something to do with it. I try to leave her alone." Both children and their parents were aware of the problems in their relationship, with parents also noticing changes in their children's behavior. Children who experienced conflict with their parent were more withdrawn, with higher levels of anxiety and depression. They also showed more aggression and acting-out behavior as well as an increase in accidents.

Mothers reported tension with their children more than did fathers during the first year after the loss. This is interesting, as fathers generally had greater difficulty adapting to the role of a single parent. "My mother took on some of the things that my father used to do. She got stricter," said a boy in his early teens. Another teenage boy reported, "My mother and I argue a lot. She never admits she's wrong. I can't express feelings to her. She doesn't understand me." High levels of parent–child conflict were likely to persist, but by the second year, mothers no longer experienced more tension than fathers. Adolescent girls were now perceived as creating the most tension, but that could be a function of their ages (72% of the girls were in the teen category at 2 years). Conflict in the family was more likely when the surviving parent was depressed, and when the family was larger, less cohesive, and experiencing more concurrent changes and stressors.

At 2 years after the death, children were more optimistic about their relationships with their surviving parent than were the parents themselves. Child-defined positive relationships were more likely when children were younger and when the surviving parent was a mother. Preteen boys were most likely to report the relationship as good, while adolescents living with fathers were least likely to report a good relationship.

Many children (59%), however, were still concerned about the safety of their surviving parent at 2 years. These children also worried about how the family would manage and tried to be "good," both to please the dead parent and to avoid adding to their surviving parent's burden by being "bad." "It's like I have to take care of Mummy. She can take care of herself, but I have to sort of give her encouragement and say, 'Oh great, Mom, you're jogging today.' I do more chores because if I don't do them, she has to. I try not to give her too many problems which is, you know, what a grown up does," said an 11-year-old girl. Her 15-year-old sister also felt some of this same responsibility: "It's hard knowing I have to take care of Mommy a little bit. Before it was, like, Daddy would come home and it would be fine. Now I will ask her if she is okay." Reflecting their need to be good, these children showed the lowest levels of aggression and delinquent behavior on the CBCL.

CHANGES IN DAILY LIFE

The death of a parent brings about inevitable changes in the daily life of the children, and change is another important mediator of responses to loss. Previous studies have indicated a positive effect on bereavement adjustment when fewer daily life changes are experienced by the children (Reese, 1982). The longer changes and disruptions in daily life continued, the greater the impact they appeared to have on the children in the Child Bereavement Study. What were the changes that these children experienced?

Four Months after the Death

During the early months after the loss, the most frequent changes concerned chores and household duties, as various roles and responsibilities were reallocated among family members: "We never had to do chores before because my mother would be home all day. Now he leaves us a piece of paper telling us what to do." Many of the children (44%) reported changes in daily chores. As might be expected, older children were most likely to be involved in such changes.

The next most frequent change experienced by children was the shifting of rooms and sleeping arrangements. These changes were more likely to occur after a sudden death or when the child had lost a parent of the opposite gender. Preteen girls were most affected in this regard and preteen boys least affected. Several of the mothers shared a bed with their children in the early months after the death. Some children also experienced changes in bed-time hours. "Before, I would go to bed at 9:30, now it's 11:30 on school nights, and I almost fall asleep sometimes in school. When I say, 'I'm going to bed,' my father says, 'Already? It's early,'" reported a 13-year-old girl. Another teenage girl who was also living with her father said, "If I was, like, up real late doing homework, Mom would make me go to bed and get up early the next day. With my father he'll just let me stay up till I finish and just go to bed."

Mealtime changes were more frequent after the death of a mother, clearly reflecting the difficulties many fathers experienced in becoming single parents. However, changes in financial status and in parents' working arrangements were more likely to occur after a father's death. In some cases the death of a parent resulted in financial difficulties and children's allowances had to be cut. "Before Dad died, I used to get a weekly allowance but now I just ask for money," said a 13-year-old girl. Some older children needed to find employment to help the family financially. This work was usually part-time and did not interfere with school responsibilities.

Overall, we found that children who experienced the greatest number of changes during the first 4 months after the death were those who lost a mother and, for these children, this also resulted in an increase in family arguments. Contrary to our expectations, high change scores during this period were not associated with more emotional/behavioral disturbance, other than an increase in children's health problems.

First-Year Changes

Changes continued to increase slightly during the first year of bereavement, but not to a significant degree. During this time, additional children experienced changes in mealtimes, and in bedtime and room arrangements. Many still reported new or different household responsibilities, as well as changes in financial status. "I used to eat supper and then go out but now I help my dad by watching my sister while he cleans up," a 10-year-old boy told us. It is interesting to note that the death of a mother no longer led to the greatest number of changes as it had in the early months.

It was only now, a year after the death, that changes in the children's daily routines were beginning to affect their behavior in significant ways. For example, changes in room arrangements and in bedtime hours primarily affected younger children and were associated with difficulties in concentration and with learning problems. These same children also saw themselves as less competent in school than their peers. Additional household responsibilities, especially for girls, reduced the amount of free time and time spent with friends. These added responsibilities, which may have been more graciously accepted around the time of the death, were more likely to be resented as the children moved through their first year of bereavement.

Second-Year Changes

During the second year of bereavement, changes in daily life activities continued, but the number of total overall changes was not significantly different from that experienced by nonbereaved counterparts. Half the children, mostly adolescents, had experienced some change in allowance and employment, and many of the same children worried about how their family would manage financially.

Shifts in household responsibilities were fewer and frequently affected girls. It is interesting to note that shifts in chores and household responsibilities were still ongoing 2 years after the death of a mother, but less so after the death of a father. Exemplifying this was a comment by a girl who was 15: "The most difficult thing during these past 2 years is trying to get used to being the only female around the house—cleaning and doing all the chores and everything. When my brothers are fighting . . . I go in my room and start thinking about my mother, what she would do. I'm still angry at my mother 'cause she left all this responsibility." It is of interest that this same girl keeps her mother's wedding ring hidden in her bedroom. The number of mealtime changes at 2 years were fewer, but these were still greater in number than those experienced by the nonbereaved group. Children who reported the greatest number of changes during the second year of bereavement reported more arguments in the family and poorer relationships between themselves and their surviving parent. "I cry when my dad makes me clean up my room. It's a mess. When she was around, she would help me," said a 12-year-old boy. Although children with many second-year changes did not report more learning problems, they continued to see themselves as performing worse in school than their peers. They also tended to be highly attached to their deceased parent—dreaming about him or her, feeling watched, prizing mementos, and wanting to behave well for the deceased's benefit.

Although daily life changes affected the children's behavior in various ways, the number of changes experienced by *the family as a whole,* assessed by the FILE (McCubbin et al., 1979), had a more significant impact on the children. This is related, in part, to the fact that a greater number of family changes was associated with parental depression. The combination of a depressed parent, a large number of family changes, and a parent with a passive coping style increased the likelihood of a child experiencing emotional and behavioral difficulties and ending up in the at-risk group (see Chapter 6).

CHANGES IN COMMUNICATION PATTERNS

One way to facilitate the grief process is to talk about the deceased and the circumstances of the death (Worden, 1991). Families varied in their ability to do this. In the early months after the loss, two-thirds of the children reported frequent family conversations about the deceased and said that they were able to share their grief within the family. This left a third of the children with fewer opportunities to talk and share feelings of grief.

Such communication was often initiated by the surviving parent. "My mom's not just letting it go. I cry and talk to Mom. I don't ignore it. I figured this out when I'd get mad from keeping it in," said a 10-year-old girl. "With Mom I can sometimes talk about my feelings and sometimes we talk about Dad, what he was like and what it would be like if he were here," revealed a 13-year-old girl.

Sometimes communication was indirectly initiated. "I usually feel sad because I can tell Dad is sad by the change of his voice, like he gets, you know, softer and then I know we can both be sad together. My dad loved her also so I guess he knows what I am going through. We are both going through the same things and he understands," said an 11-year-old girl.

Some children expressed discomfort when the surviving parent would bring up a discussion of the deceased. "My father says, 'Do you miss your mother?' and things like that. He keeps reminding us that Mother's not around, and he acts like we don't realize she's dead. He thinks we take life as it comes. He keeps talking about it all the time and I just change the subject or something," said a 17-year-old boy. His 13-year-old sister felt unsatisfied with the family communication because she was the only girl in the family: "If the family was complete, I'd know that there's someone else there to talk to besides my father. The worse thing is not having this; it's all male in my family—all males." In another family an 11-year-old girl was prompted to talk by her mother: "Mom asks me a lot, like what I miss about him the most and if I feel anything different, but I really don't. I feel like I know that he's gone but I don't feel like I'm a different person, a whole new different person." Her brother, age 10, found the mother's prompting helpful: "I talk to my mother. We say that we love him still; just because he's dead doesn't mean we can't love him still."

Some children felt more comfortable speaking with friends or a sibling rather than their surviving parent. "I talk to my friends and also to my younger brother. He knows what I'm talking about when we talk. I don't talk with my mother," said a 16-year-old boy. There were other children who never spoke with their siblings about the dead parent. "I don't talk to my brother. We don't ever talk about it. It's like a closed topic," stated another adolescent. He also said, "Once in a while Mom tries to get me to talk about it, but I really don't like to. I just think it out for myself." Another teenage boy said, "I don't talk to her about it if it's at all possible. She doesn't need to be worried about me."

At 1 year children who had lost mothers had the most difficulty talking about their dead parent and were also having more emotional/behavioral problems. These children also had difficulty speaking to peers about the deceased. The child's age and gender were not significantly related to this difficulty.

At this point the majority of children (78%) felt that they had adequate opportunity to talk about the deceased parent within the family, usually daily or at least several times a week. Many of the children in these families were still attached to the deceased, and the majority were able to share their dreams of the lost parent with another family member.

It is interesting that families in which the deceased could be discussed openly were not always those with the highest functioning parents. Although these conversations were more likely to take place in cohesive families, some surviving parents in these families reported high levels of depression as well as intrusive and avoidant thinking. Conversations about the deceased were more likely to take place in families in which the mother was the surviving parent.

At 1 year 30% of the children were seen by the parent as having difficulty talking about the deceased, similar to the percentage who had difficulty talking 4 months after the death. By 2 years after the death, fewer children had difficulty speaking of the dead parent, although 23% of the children still found it hard to do so, as did this girl who was 10 when her father died: "I don't mention my father 'cause I don't want to see her cry. She is always telling me to talk about it. If I talk about it, it will be better. I just don't want to talk about it!" At 2 years, a significantly large proportion (54%) of children who still dreamed about the dead parent were able to share these dreams with another family member. Children generally felt most comfortable speaking to the surviving parent, followed by their siblings.

THE CHILD'S RELATIONSHIP WITH PEERS

The majority of children reported having two or more friends, and this number did not change significantly over the 2 years of bereavement. Neither were there significant changes in social activities when the bereaved children were compared to their nonbereaved counterparts. In the early months after the death, a fifth of the children reported spending more time with friends than before the death. These were often children who had experienced the sudden loss of a parent. A few children spent less time. "I spend less time with my friend. I get depressed and stay home," said an 11-year-old boy.

For some children, having only one parent created a sense of stigma. When possible, these children preferred to hide the fact that one of their parents is dead. An 8-year-old girl reflected this concern when she said, "I don't like to talk to other kids about this because I don't want them to tease me."

A small group of children in the early months after the death (14%) said they were given a bad time by peers for not having both parents. These tended to be younger children, in many cases, preteen girls. The number of children being teased dropped (9%) during the first year, but remained constant at the second assessment, with mostly the same children reporting this phenomenon. Teasing took the form of taunting the bereaved child. "Ha ha, you don't have a mother and I do," said a neighbor child to one 12-year-old girl. "How's the stiff doing?" was the taunt of children to two boys whose father had died. "How's your mother doing? Oh, sorry, I forgot," was a comment frequently addressed to another child. As one 11-year-old girl told us of this bullying behavior, she broke down sobbing: "I tell them, 'I don't have a father. Could you stop being mean to me, 'cause I'm having a hard time.' "

We asked children if they were embarrassed or felt "different" because of the death. At 1 year one-third of the children reported feeling this way. One young girl said that she didn't want to talk about the loss because she did not want her friends to treat her differently. Several of the children said they did not want to be pitied by other children. These feelings were most likely to be experienced by adolescents, particularly older adolescent girls. Children were also asked whether other children understood how it felt to lose a parent to death. Nearly half the children reported a lack of understanding, with this response coming from boys and girls of all ages.

In the early months after the death, half of the children were talking to friends about the death. These were more likely to be girls, especially adolescent girls; those talking least were boys, especially preteen boys. Children who were able to talk with the surviving parent at home were more likely to be talking with friends.

There were a number of reasons given by the children for *not* speaking with their friends about the death of their parent. Some of these are as follows:

1. *Fear of crying in front of friends.* A 12-year-old boy who didn't talk to his friends about his mother's death explained, " 'Cause I'd start crying in front of them. I don't want to cry. 'Cause I get headaches when I cry." "When playing sports I try not to cry in

front of my friends. I don't want them making fun of me," said a 10-year-old boy whose father died.

2. *The subject never arises.* "I never talk to my friends. It never comes up," reported a 13-year-old boy who lost his father. A girl who was 11 when her mother died said, "I don't talk to them about it unless they say anything. They used to but not anymore." "My friends think I should be over it. They don't say it; it's just the way they look at me," noted a teenage girl who was 11 when her mother died.

3. *Friends are protective of the bereaved child.* A year after the death one 11-year-old girl said, "If I say, 'This is what my father got me,' they think if they keep talking about it, I'll get sad because in the past I've gotten sad talking about it. They just don't want me to get sad. I just want them to listen. I can't blame them because they never had their father die." "My friends don't talk because they know it makes me sad, and I doubt that they even feel comfortable," explained a teenage boy whose dad died. "Kids at school try not to talk about it that much. They just, like, act normally, play games at recess, so, like, it wouldn't bother me," a 12-year-old boy told us.

4. *Awkwardness on the part of friends.* "Like, they know my father had died but I don't think they knew how to act," said one preteen girl. "Two people in my class asked me what happened maybe a week afterward. One asked me, 'Do you like talking about your father?' I said, 'Yeah,' and that was it," said another preteen girl.

5. *Not knowing about the death.* "Most of my friends don't know about my father," reported a 9-year-old girl, 2 years after the death of her dad. It could be awkward when friends were not informed of the death. One 13-year-old girl attended a sleepover with some girlfriends. "Where's your father been? Are your parents divorced or something?" her friends asked. Afterward these girls felt bad when they found out.

6. *Not caring.* An 11-year-old boy said, "I don't talk to friends about my mother. I guess they don't really care. They're interested more in sports than in listening to me."

7. *Circumstances of the death.* A 6-year-old girl whose father committed suicide revealed, "I've never told them that he died 'cause they would tell everyone else and then they will ask me about the death." After 2 years, this girl had been able to share the

circumstances of her father's death with a friend. In this same interview she made the telling comment, "I was almost 6 when he died, now I'm 8 and wiser."

8. *Feels too personal.* "With my friends it never comes up. We're too busy with other stuff. I wouldn't like to. It's my business and it's not a nice thing. It would upset me and my friends," asserted a teenage boy. One 15-year-old girl said, "In school I don't want everybody knowing my business. I don't tell them nothing!"

A few things made it easier for bereaved children to speak with their friends. One was having a friend who had gone through a similar loss. "I have a friend who lost his father and he knows what it was like going through," said a 10-year-old boy whose father died. Even having a friend from a divorced family made communication easier. A 13-year-old boy told us that the one who understands him best is a friend who lives with his divorced father. Having older friends also helped with communication. One teenage boy found it easier to speak about his dad with an older friend who brings up the subject. "He says, 'I remember your father used to love doing this or that,' and I agree with him." This same boy found it difficult to discuss the father's death with his 16-year-old brother even though he said that they were close. For some children it was easier to communicate with a friend who knew the deceased parent. A 10-year-old boy found it easiest to talk with a friend who knew his mother. "We really remind each other of memories," he said with some enthusiasm. There were several older teenage boys who had difficulty speaking with peers until they met a new girlfriend who made it easier for them to talk. "At first I felt overwhelming sadness but then I shut myself off. This has changed since my new girlfriend," expressed a 17-year-old.

During the first and second years of bereavement, the number of children talking with friends about the death remained about the same. Those who had been talking continued to do so, while those who weren't talking were not likely to begin at this point. Curiously, there was a small group of six children who did not want to talk about their parent but who had friends who wanted to talk about the loss. Children who were communicating with peers were more connected to the dead parent and had higher levels of self-esteem and self-efficacy than those children who were not communicating with friends.

Being with peers who had two living parents often brought out strong feelings in the bereaved children. "I am reminded constantly that they have it made because they have a father," said an 11-year-old girl whose father died. One friend with two parents told a 6-year-old boy, "You're lucky you don't have a father." Although intended to be helpful, the comment made the child feel very sad. "You hear kids, like, say they hate their parents and stuff. It's like you don't know how much you like them until you lose them," was the sad comment from a 16-year-old boy who lost his father. A teenage boy felt uncomfortable with his friends saying, "Can't your mother take us?" and then after realizing what they've said, rephrasing the statement, "Oh, I mean your father." "When I visit their home, I sometimes wonder when I see their father what things would be like with my father and stuff like that. How would my life be different if my father were here. How would my parents get along? What would my friends think of him? I can't piece it together, how it would be like," said a 14-year-old boy. "My girlfriend talks about her father. Friends take it for granted that they have a father. If they could see what it is like, they might be a little more understanding," asserted a 16-year-old boy 2 years after his dad's death. "Other kids talk about their fathers, 'My father does this or that.' It just makes me feel like I am left out, like I am missing something," revealed a teenage boy. A 10-year-old girl admitted, "When I get mad it's usually because my friends have fathers. Maybe I'm a little bit jealous that they have fathers. I don't get mad at friends whose parents are divorced even though they still have fathers." A 17-year-old boy said, "When they start talking about their parents, I kind of feel left out sometimes."

Two years after the death, social problems and changes in social self-perception began to surface. At that time, bereaved children had *more* social problems than their nonbereaved counterparts, as perceived both by their parents (as per the CBCL) and themselves (as per Harter's [1979] Perceived Competence Scale for Children). An 11-year-old girl told us, "A few times when we're at the school, I'll start crying because everyone will have, like, two parents or they've divorced them. But I don't have my dad. It's real hard to go to school; kids don't know how to react. I don't know; it's hard to be around them. I can't talk to them." Children with social problems were more likely to be concerned about their own safety, to feel less in control over events in their lives, and to have lower self-esteem. It should be noted that these difficulties were associated more with the death of a mother than of a father.

THE CHILD'S RELATIONSHIP WITH TEACHERS

Nearly all of the teachers were informed of the death, and 42% of them made an announcement to the child's class. These announcements were not always well received by the bereaved child. "My teacher was reading short stories of Poe and said to that class that we might have to stop when I came back because it might be too gruesome or scary to go on reading it. I felt totally ridiculous, and I was so embarrassed," said a 15-year-old girl. Her younger brother had a more positive reaction to his teacher's announcement: "My teacher had a father who died during the summer. She brought it up in class that me and her might have a harder Christmas than the rest of the kids." A mixed review came from an 11-year-old boy whose teacher "told the kids to go easy on me, so they don't call me names anymore. It's boring somehow."

One-third of the children wanted to talk about the death with their teachers and the teachers were willing to comply. Another third of the children were not interested in talking and their teachers did not initiate conversations about the death. The rest of the children, mainly adolescent boys, reported that their teachers wanted to speak with them about the death, but they were reluctant to do so. A 13-year-old girl found a creative way to end attempts at communication by teachers: "I just tell them in school that I can't talk to them without my mother's permission. So that's been getting them away." Her 14-year-old brother also did not want to talk to his eager teachers: "It's just my feelings, and if I want to talk to them, I will. I just don't want them trying to go down and take them out." A similar sentiment was expressed by a girl who was 15 when her father died: "The school should keep out of it mostly. They are never involved with you, and then they suddenly come in when something awful happens, it's like vultures."

There were only two children who reported discomfort on the teacher's part. All in all, it seemed that teachers were available and willing to talk about the loss with the children. Some teachers were especially sensitive to the needs of the children. An 11-year-old girl whose mother died said, "Usually my teacher can see, like, water come in my eyes and she will pull me in the hall and ask me what's the matter. I tell her and she tells me she wants me to go down to the lavatory. I go, think it over, and go back in and finish my school work."

As time passed and children were promoted to other classes, some new teachers were not aware of the death. One teenage boy had an awkward moment: "In school we were talking about family trees and they asked, 'What is your mother's name?' I can't really say my mother is dead so I just said it, pretending that she was still alive. No one is going to know."

POINTS TO REMEMBER:
HOW LIFE CHANGES

- Three things that children need after the death of a parent are support, nurturance, and continuity. Providing these may be difficult for a surviving parent, particularly for a surviving father.
- Physical and emotional availability of the surviving parent are important to the child's adjustment to loss. Bereaved mothers are often more available for their children than are bereaved fathers.
- When bereavement leads to depression in the surviving parent, such parents may be less aware of their children's needs.
- Some children become closer to their surviving parent after a death while others experience high levels of tension. Tension is more likely if the family is large, less cohesive, and is experiencing more concurrent changes and stressors.
- Surviving parents set the tone for family conversations about the deceased; mothers tend to find this an easier task than fathers. Talking about the deceased is important to the tasks of mourning, but not talking does not necessarily lead to more emotional and behavioral difficulties.
- Changes in daily life and routine are more likely to be experienced by children who lose mothers rather than fathers,

especially in the early months after a loss. The impact of change on the child's behavior becomes greater the further out one is from the death.

• Bereaved teenagers frequently feel different than their friends because of the loss and often feel that their friends do not understand how it is to lose a parent to death.

• Social problems are more likely to show up 2 years after the death and are found more frequently in the bereaved than in their nonbereaved counterparts.

• Teachers, for the most part, are willing to discuss the death with the child if the child wants to have such discussions about the loss.

F · O · U · R

How the Child Responds

In this chapter we will look closely at how the child him- or herself is affected by the death of a parent. I will discuss the major outcome variables in the Child Bereavement Study such as the children's expressions of sadness, fear, and anger; what they think and feel about themselves; and their health and school performance.

EMOTIONAL LIFE

Affective expressions are a normal part of the bereavement process. The four expressions we saw most frequently in the children were sadness, anxiety, guilt, and anger. The latter was often expressed in acting-out behavior.

Sadness and Crying

Sadness is expected when a parent dies and the most frequent expression of sadness is crying. Most children cried on hearing of the death, and two-thirds cried again sometime during the initial weeks. By the first anniversary of the death, crying had decreased significantly; however 13% were still crying daily or weekly. Boys were the least likely to cry and girls the most likely.

There was a wide range of individual differences in the degree of crying that children displayed. Some cried very little while others seemed to be inconsolable. For some children there was an initial burst of tears but then an attempt to refrain from crying in an effort to make it easier on the surviving parent, by giving the impression that they were coping. For other children, especially boys, there was the direct or subtle message that they must now act more "grown up" because of a parent's death. Adolescent boys were most likely to say they were not crying 4 months after the death.

One-fourth of the children, mostly adolescents, were given the dictum to show *more* feeling. The mother of one 16-year-old boy pushed him to grieve more: "She tells me, 'Why are you holding onto those things? You should just let them out and stuff.' It gets boring after a while." Occasionally kids were prompted by friends to show more sadness. "My girlfriend said that I didn't seem sad enough," said one teenage girl. Adolescents, in general, had more difficulty talking about their feelings and reported feeling "strange" and "embarrassed" with peers who had not experienced the death of a parent. They also worried about how their family would manage after the loss and were more likely to fear for the safety of their surviving parent.

Crying was often triggered by the behavior of others. "I saw Mom crying and I just began crying with her," said one girl. A boy reported seeing others crying and thinking that he should cry, but then realizing that he did not feel like crying. Some cried when they thought that was expected of them. "Mom wanted me to cry a lot, so I did," stated an 11-year-old girl after her father died.

The children with the most frequent crying included those who were highly connected with the dead parent—those who often thought about, spoke to, and dreamed of the deceased. These children also tended to idealize the dead parent and to see themselves as more like this parent than the surviving one. For a few children, mostly younger, there was the belief that if they just cried hard enough, they might get the parent to return. This is understandable when one realizes that crying behavior, from the earliest days of infancy, brings a comforting response from the parent. Except for those adolescents given the dictum to act more adult, very few children in the study (3%) were told to show *less* feeling of grief.

A number of factors would trigger sadness in these children, often leading to crying. One was missing activities previously shared with the parent. "If it was something I liked doing with him, I start crying. I remember doing it and I can't do it again," said an 8-year-old boy. A similar sentiment was expressed by another 8-year-old who lost his father through a homicide: "I miss being able to do father and son things like having him at games." A 14-year-old boy felt considerable sadness when he realized that his father no longer could go fishing with him. A 13-year-old boy confided, "My dad is not here to encourage and help me with sports and school. He was very supportive." The loss of shared activities was particularly keen among boys who lost fathers, especially those who were in the preteen years.

Other children, frequently girls, felt sad over missed opportunities to show a lost parent new accomplishments. "I want her to see my report card tomorrow. I think I'm doing better than last year," said a 11-year-old girl. "I missed her on graduation. I would like to show her my diploma," said a 17-year-old boy who had not had a close relationship with his mother before her death. A 10-year-old girl told us, "I try a little harder because I want him to be proud of me, so I try a little harder every year." A similar thought was expressed by a teenage boy: "The reason I try more in all sports is 'cause I want to win for her." A young boy of 6 told us, "I want to show my father pictures that I drew. I love him. He'd like them." This same child was also aware of missing shared activities: "I want him back where I would get to see him all the time. I don't get to do stuff with him."

Sometimes sadness was comingled with regrets: "Sometimes I cry, especially in my room at night. I think about how I used to call her names. I really never told her I loved her directly." Nighttime frequently brought about sad feelings. "Sometimes I get really sad in the night and I call out to my sister," said an 8-year-old boy. His sister, age 11, also experienced most of her sadness at night: "It usually happens in the night because in the night I don't really have to think about anything. When I'm in school I have to think about what I am working on."

Others were aware that they no longer would receive advice and counsel from the dead parent and this led to sadness, and sometimes anger. "It's just, like, not having a man to help me out; so it's like being deserted. That's the worst part of losing a father," reported a 16-year-old boy. Another teenage boy expressed sadness: "I want my father here to give me advice." Similarly, a young teen boy said, "I would like my mother to be around to help me with school and help me grow up."

For most, sadness came when they realized that they no longer could share the presence or the touch of the dead parent. "I feel sad thinking that I can't see him except in pictures," reported an 11-year-old boy. "He's not here to hug me," was the sad report of a teenage girl. A 13-year-old boy was sad not for himself but for his brother who was 6: "The first week I cried; it wasn't for me, it was for my brother because of all the things I had that he wouldn't. I had a lot more time with my father than he did."

Crying decreased significantly for the children during the first year of bereavement. "My sadness has gotten less than before. I sit there and wait and try not to think about it. I don't tell my mother. I don't want to see her upset but it could be helpful to talk," said a 13-year-old girl. Around the first anniversary, 37% reported that they never cried now about the loss. Some of the children reported that they were "all cried out" and were now beyond crying. Girls were more likely to report strong feelings of sadness and frequent crying behavior 1 year after the loss, as were those who were still very connected to the dead parent.

While the overall frequency of crying decreased over time, the majority of children (66%) reported that they still cried occasionally 2 years after the death. A small group of five children, four of whom were teen girls, said the loss hurt more after 2 years than it had earlier. "It hurts more now. Earlier, people were around more. Now I feel bad and no one is there."

Anxiety

It is understandable that bereaved children might experience anxiety. In the first place, they may fear losing another loved one, especially the one remaining parent. Second, anxiety can also be associated with the child's own safety. "Will it happen to me?" is a question often asked by bereaved children. Looking at these two types of anxiety, we found that many children do feel fearful, but significantly more so a year after the death than right away. Anxiety was highly associated with an increased number of changes and disruptions in daily life, and with feeling less in control over one's circumstances. In general, anxiety was higher for girls than for boys.

At 4 months after the parent's death, we found that close to half of the children (44%) expressed fear for their surviving parent's safety. This was especially true in the case of mother loss. At 1 year after the death this fear had risen to 62%. By the second anniversary of the death, the figure had declined significantly but was still high, with half of the children expressing this fear. It may be that the reality of having only one parent became more apparent to these children as they went through the first year of loss, and this realization led to an increase in anxiety. Children's fear for their own personal safety also rose slightly over the first year from 11% to 16% and was associated with the loss of a father.

Some of the anxiety expressed by girls took the following foci: "I stay home with my mom. I guess I was scared to leave at first. Now it's better. But I always feel better when I know where she is." "I am afraid that he will get hit and killed on the bicycle that he rides to work." "If she dies, then I wouldn't know what was going to happen. And I wouldn't like it anywhere I lived besides here." "It worries me when Mother comes home late from work and she doesn't tell me." "Well, I don't want Mummy to die because that would leave me with a lot of stuff to do, and I want to get to go off to college and be a grown-up; and if she dies, then I'll have to take care of everybody completely, forever."

Boys also expressed anxiety over the surviving parent's safety. Here are some examples: "I worry about my father getting into a car accident and dying. Where will we go?" "On New Year's Eve, she went out and was home very late. I was worried and wanted to yell at her." "I am afraid when she yells and stuff that she might get a heart attack and then I will be an orphan." "I was afraid when she went on a plane to Mexico." "I had a dream that something bad happened to my father. I had to take care of the family myself. I couldn't possibly pay for anything and I couldn't handle college and all at the same time. My father told me not to worry, it was just a dream."

The effects of smoking on their surviving parent's health gave some children concern. A 13-year-old girl expressed this: "I am worried about my mother's health. When she coughs because she smokes, I want to make her stop smoking. I'd like to throw these [cigarettes on table beside the interviewer] out the door." "I am concerned about my father and asked him to stop smoking," reported another child.

Some children expressed concern over the functioning of the family now that there was only one parent. "She used to bring money home, and I thought that my father wouldn't be able to buy us, like, clothes and the stuff we need," expressed a 13-year-old boy. Another teenage boy asked his mother if she was going back to work because he thought they would "like, go broke or something." He was reassured by his mother that they were "all set." Another boy feared that "nothing would be organized after Mother died. Things would kinda fall apart." Girls also expressed such concern for family functioning. "I worried when my father went to work at night that there would be no one to help me," shared a girl in her early teens, even though she had two older siblings. Another girl worried about "if Mom would be able to support us and if we would have to sell this house." Still another girl wondered how her mother would manage with four kids.

Which children tended to be more fearful? We had anticipated that a child's fear for the parent's safety would be greater when the deceased parent had a sudden or unnatural death (suicide, accident, or homicide), but such was not the case. Greater fear for the surviving parent's safety was found in children whose parent died of natural causes. One possible explanation is that the observation of a parent in a deteriorating condition brought home the reality of dying and death in a way that was not present if the death was sudden.

Over time, the profile of the most fearful children shifted somewhat. At 4 months after the death, preteen girls expressed the most fear, boys the least. When anxiety peaked at 1 year, fear was highest for adolescent girls and lowest for adolescent boys. More fear was also found in children who lost an opposite-gender parent (girls losing fathers or boys losing mothers).

During the second year after the death, girls continued to be the most fearful, with twice as many girls as boys fearful of their surviving parent's safety. Girls who were preadolescent at the time of the parent's death tended to be the most fearful. "I am still worried about Mother," confided a girl 2 years after the death of her father when she was 6. "At night I think she stops breathing.

I worry every night." Children who felt less good about them-selves and who had less peer support were more fearful, as were children with more social problems and less sense of control over their circumstances.

Children who feared for their own personal safety were more likely to believe that their dead parent was just "away" and would be returning at some point—a belief that caused them *not* to think of the parent in a specific place such as heaven. These same children also reported being told by family members that they were not grieving sufficiently and that they should be grieving more.

Guilt

It is common for survivors to feel guilt after the death of a loved one, and this was true for some of these children. Guilt usually took the form of regrets for things done or not done—apologies not extended or affection not expressed. "I always used to talk back to my mother and I never got a chance to say, 'I'm sorry,' " said a boy who was 11 when his mother died. He still bore regrets 2 years later when he sobbed, saying, "I never said, 'I love you' to her. Now I wish she could be back and I could say it. Maybe when she died she didn't know that I loved her. I didn't want her dying thinking that." His brother, 17, harbored similar regrets: "I really never told her I loved her, directly." Their 15-year-old brother was also remorseful: "I would have told her I was sorry for the things I did." The only child in this family with no regrets was the sister, who was 13 at the time of death. She told her mother that she loved her while her mother was still in a coma. After that her mother moved so she thought that the mother had heard her.

Similar expressions of guilt were expressed by a girl who was 9 when her father died. After 2 years had passed, she said, "I still feel guilty. I wanted to say things to him that I should have said, like how much I cared for him, that I didn't want him to leave." Some children regretted the lack of time spent with the parent before the illness and death. "I feel guilty over not having quality time together," said a 17-year-old boy. "I can't change what already happened. I didn't spend enough time with him. After they are gone, they are gone. Maybe if I had said, 'I love you' to him. I never said it." Others expressed regrets over the way they inter-

acted with the parent around the time of death. "Part of me thinks
that I should have stayed with him at the hospital the whole last
day. It wouldn't have made a difference to the outcome but part
of me thinks that it would," confided a 17-year-old boy. One
14-year-old boy still felt guilty regarding his father's health 2 years
after the death: "I still feel guilty, maybe I should have said more
to him, like watching his health." Of interest was a 6-year-old girl
whose father committed suicide. She did not assume any responsibility, as sometimes happens after a suicidal death: "It was his own
fault. He killed himself."

Anger and Acting-Out Behavior

Some bereaved children, especially boys, have been observed to
express their feelings of grief through anger and acting-out behavior (Black, 1978). Feelings of abandonment often underly such
anger. Elizur and Kaffman (1982) found high levels of aggressive
behavior in their longitudinal study of bereaved Israeli children
who lost fathers during the Yom Kippur War. Children in the Child
Bereavement Study did show higher levels of aggression than their
nonbereaved counterparts. This was especially true 1 year after the
death of the parent. "I get angry. He was too young to die, too
nice a person to die," said a 14-year-old boy about his father.

Children directed their anger toward various targets. Some
were angry with God. "I am angry at God for taking him away,"
said a 9-year-old boy 2 years after his father died. A 12-year-old
boy who arrived at the hospital too late to see his dying mother
cried at the hospital and then went home and punched his
punching bag: "At first I got really angry. I was mad at God that
he took my mom. Now I don't get as angry. I just feel depressed."
Others were angry at the parent for dying and leaving them. "I'm
angry at him for leaving and putting us through this. I feel that
it's his place to care for others," said a boy in his early teens. An
11-year-old boy was still mad at his father 2 years after the death:
"I'm mad that he's dead and that I didn't know him for long."

The children who showed more aggressive behavior over the
2-year period were also more fearful of the safety of their surviving
parent, were less able to speak of their dead parent within the family
or with friends, and had a lower sense of self-efficacy. These

characteristics are consistent with the idea that children may externalize their internal conflicts through acting-out behavior. It may be that such behavior was a means of getting a strong reaction from the surviving parent, as well as giving the child a greater sense of empowerment. For example, a 10-year-old girl, whose anger and acting-out behavior began during her father's illness, increased her acting out after his death. This behavior resulted in a major change in the mother's work routine. This girl also experienced considerable anxiety when her mother became ill after the death and had to be hospitalized.

Sometimes a family member believed that a child should feel anger when, in fact, the child wasn't feeling any. "My uncle said that it was alright if I felt angry, but I didn't feel any anger at all. I sort of think if your father dies suddenly you'd be angry but if it's long term, then you know it's going to happen. But I was really sad," said a preteen girl whose father had died after a lengthy illness.

Delinquent behavior was clearly related to mother loss and was more likely to be found in adolescents than preadolescents. At both the 1- and 2-year assessments, this behavior was found most frequently in the group of girls who were adolescents when their mothers died. This unusual finding could be due to a number of factors. The fathers' expectations of these girls were high. Often, as the oldest females in the family, they took on the responsibility for care of the younger children and management of the household. "I was angry at my mother 'cause she left me all this responsibility. I'm still angry!" asserted a girl who was 13 when her mother died. Another contributing factor relates to developmental issues. These girls were deprived of the presence of their mothers in early adolescence, a time during which a close relationship with the same-sex parent is of particular importance. For example, psycho-analysts believe that early oedipal conflicts are resolved through identification with the same-gender parent. When this same-gen-der parent is missing from the family, such a resolution is more difficult and the resulting internal conflicts may lead to acting-out behavior. Finally, fathers were more likely than mothers to be dating during this period, and the introduction of a new female into the home could add stress, leading to acting-out behavior.

Aggressive and delinquent behaviors were more common in families where the surviving parent, regardless of gender, was

functioning less well. These types of problem behaviors are correlated with high levels of parental stress and depression, along with
the parent's use of less effective coping strategies, low family
cohesion, more younger children, high levels of family change, and
fewer financial resources.

HEALTH STATUS

Health problems have been identified as a possible consequence of
bereavement in adults, and there has been an interest in this
phenomenon in bereaved children (Osterweis et al., 1984). In the
Child Bereavement Study we looked closely at children's health
issues, especially in the areas of somaticization, illnesses, and accidents. Somaticization and health problems were found more
frequently in the bereaved group than the control group, especially
during the first year after the parent's death. Girls tended to
experience these problems more often than boys.

Somaticization

Somaticization as an expression of grief in bereaved children has
been of interest to researchers, especially the experience of headaches and stomachaches (Sood et al., 1992). E. Furman (1974) has
hypothesized that younger children, who have more limited verbal
abilities, tend to somaticize more than older children or adults in
response to a loss.

In the early months after the death, a fifth of the children
experienced frequent headaches, with a larger percentage of girls
reporting these headaches than boys: "I just get headaches a lot and
I never got them before." Thirteen percent of the children
manifested somatic symptoms in the clinical range on the somatic
scale of the CBCL at this time. These symptoms were more
frequently experienced by preteen children and by children who
had lost a father. Although children in the matched nonbereaved
control group experienced a similar percentage of headaches, only
4% of this group had somatic scores in the clinical range.

Levels of somaticization continued without significant reduction during the first year of bereavement. Higher levels of somatic

symptoms were most likely to be found in children whose families experienced a large number of disruptions after the death. These children were anxious about their own safety, had problems with peer relationships, and felt some culpability about the death of their parent.

During the second year of bereavement, 17% of the children continued to experience frequent headaches. This is not a significant reduction from the first year, nor is it appreciably different from the percentage experienced by the matched nonbereaved controls. Again, headaches were more frequent for girls, and for those children who reported good relationships with the lost parent before the death and were highly connected afterward. By this time, somatic scores in the clinical range had dropped from 13% to 8%, closer to the range found in the control group. Preteen children had the highest somatic scores, in keeping with E. Furman's (1974) hypothesis that younger children somatize more.

These somatic symptoms can be problematic for the children but they do not necessarily reflect an illness. We were also interested to discover whether or not grieving children might suffer from more illnesses as a part of their overall bereavement.

Illnesses

Although 61% of the children in the study had some type of mild illness in the 4 months after the death, only 4% suffered serious illness. Boys were as likely as girls to fall ill, but illness was more frequent among younger children. Children were more likely to suffer some type of illness when they had lost a father, and when they were experiencing more daily life changes and higher levels of conflict in the home. "I had his symptoms. I have myself convinced that I probably had the same thing," said a 10-year-old girl whose mother had also gotten sick right after the father died. As expected, sick children were most likely to be cared for by their surviving parent, although fathers often relinquished this duty to someone else.

By the end of the first year of bereavement there was a significant *increase* in the number of children who experienced a serious illness, with 10% of children reporting such an illness and four children needing hospitalization. Bereaved children were more likely than their nonbereaved counterparts to become seriously ill. Slightly more adolescent boys reported serious illnesses, but these occurred among children of both sexes and all ages. Milder illnesses were reported by 70% of the children, most often by preteen girls.

The number of serious illnesses dropped slightly to 8% during the second year of bereavement, with younger children being most likely to become ill. At this point, the percentage of serious illnesses among bereaved children was now no different than that found among nonbereaved control children.

Accidents

Under normal circumstances it is expected that certain children will experience some type of accident related to their daily lives and activities. When accidents are experienced by bereaved children, however, they may be interpreted as grief-related behavior, and this adds to the speculation as to why some bereaved children experience accidents. A common theory has to do with self-punishment. Children who feel guilty after the death of a parent may experience more accidents than those who do not feel this culpability. Another speculation has to do with getting the deceased parent to return. When a child is hurt, a parent comes to rescue the child, to apply first aid and comfort. A bereaved child may unconsciously get hurt in order to evoke the presence of the deceased parent.

In the Child Bereavement Study we found that 25% of the children, the majority being adolescent boys, experienced some type of accident in the early months following the death. Children who lost mothers were more likely to get hurt than those who lost fathers. However, only nine children, both boys and girls, had serious accidents requiring medical attention.

Those children who had some type of accident were anxious, felt personally unsafe, and were uneasy coming to the dinner table without both parents. They also tended to show more disturbed behavior, such as social withdrawal, attention seeking, and aggressive and delinquent behavior.

There was a significant *increase* in the percentage of children experiencing accidents as they moved through the first year of bereavement (34%), affecting more boys than girls. This percentage was slightly higher than the percentage of accidents experienced by nonbereaved control children (26%). Again, adolescent boys had the majority of accidents, with 45% reporting accidents and a third of these needing medical attention. More accidents were reported in households with higher levels of conflict. Children who got hurt saw themselves more as being like their deceased parent than their surviving parent and reported that they sometimes mimicked the behavior of their dead parent. These same children saw themselves as behaving less well than their peers.

By the second year bereaved children reported fewer accidents than the year before (26%) and the frequency of accidents was similar to that of the nonbereaved children. Bereaved children with accidents at this point in time felt personally less safe and were also seen to have more self-blame and regrets over the death.

SCHOOL PERFORMANCE

In the early months after their parent's death, a fifth of the children reported experiencing some type of learning difficulty in school, and a similar percentage reported difficulty in concentration. Concentration problems often arose when children were preoccupied with thoughts of their dead parent. "It is hard to sit still in class and concentrate. The words 'Dad is dead' are ringing in my ear," said one young boy. Another boy admitted, "I have difficulty concentrating 'cause, like, I always daydream about my mom and then I get all nervous about it." Still another boy of similar age reported, "Well, sometimes I'll, like, drift away when we're taking notes or something. I'll, like, drift away from the subject and think about my dad."

Boys, in general, were more likely to experience academic difficulties than girls in the early months after the death. Adolescent boys, in particular, were the most vulnerable group for learning problems. Children with fewer friends, and children whose grief manifested in sleep disturbance, headaches, and frequent crying found it difficult to concentrate. Those who had experienced mother loss were more likely to have learning difficulties at 4 months than those who lost fathers. One can speculate that it is often a mother's role to check on the child's progress in school and that mothers are more likely to be the ones to encourage the child to do homework. An 11-year-old girl said, "Mother helped me with my school work before she got sick. Well, it wasn't the help but the fact that she was gone. School is harder just knowing that she is gone. I'm not doing too well in school. I'm not doing as good as I was before she. . . . My grades are getting lower. In school I am thinking about my mother rather than the subjects." One teen boy said, "I know I could do better in school but there's no one to help me at home." Missing fathers also contributed to learning problems for some children. A 15-year-old girl said at the 1-year interview, "Last year my grades were terrible because he used to test me, to help me study, and he wasn't there to do that anymore. I wouldn't study partly because I didn't know how without help and partly because when I studied alone I kind of missed him." Her younger sister, age 11, was also having school difficulties. "Mummy will go out on the weeknights and I'll have to babysit. So I don't get started with my homework until, like, 10. Sometimes I just sit at my desk, spaced out, thinking about Daddy but I just sit there for, like, an hour. My homework is open and I don't do it."

Interestingly a small group of 22 children reported that their school work changed for the better 4 months after the death, with girls more likely to report this positive change.

As the first year of bereavement progressed, boys improved in their school performance while teenage girls began to perform worse and also began to have more concentration problems. At the first year assessment, 15% of the bereaved children had learning difficulties, down only slightly from the earlier 21%. However, this figure was no different than the percentage of nonbereaved children having such learning difficulties. Therefore, one must be cautious not to conclude, as some have (Berlinsky & Biller, 1982), that children develop more learning difficulty as a consequence of bereavement. However, there were some differences between bereaved and control children in terms of their ability to concentrate. Although concentration improved significantly for bereaved children during the first year after the death, 16% still had problems as compared to only 6% of the control children—a significant difference.

Anxiety was a strong correlate of learning difficulties at 1 year, along with uneasiness at the dinner table, headaches, and sleep problems. Children doing poorly in school at this time also had lower self-esteem, less sense of self-empowerment, higher levels of aggressive behavior, and were experiencing a larger number of changes in their daily lives.

There was a slight reduction in learning problems during the second year of bereavement, as well as some improvement in concentration. At this point, adolescents were experiencing the most learning difficulties. Those experiencing learning problems at this time cried more, had ongoing sleep problems, and continued to feel worse about themselves and their ability to control events in their lives. Again, however, there were no significant differences when comparing the frequency of learning problems of the bereaved with their nonbereaved counterparts.

SELF-PERCEPTION

A person's self-perception can have a profound effect on the way in which that person sees and interacts with the world. In turn, these interactions affect the way in which the person sees him- or herself. How the children in the study saw themselves determined, in part, how they coped with the death of their parent. Likewise, the death of their parent affected these children's perceptions of themselves. We looked at the children's evaluations of themselves in several areas, paying particular attention to the child's sense of self-efficacy, self-esteem, and sense of maturity.

Self-Efficacy

Self-efficacy, also referred to as "locus of control," is a person's perceived ability to affect and change what is happening to him or her, as opposed to feeling controlled by fate or other outside influences. There is an age-related effect for this hypothetical construct: Older children, when compared to younger, are more likely to believe they can control what happens to them (Nowicki & Strickland, 1973).

We found that bereaved children believed they were less able to effect change than their nonbereaved counterparts. This was true 1 year after the death and even more so at 2 years. Because these children were matched for age, gender, grade in school, family religion, and community, it is difficult to avoid the supposition that this difference had something to do with the death of their parent.

During the first year of bereavement, the children's sense of control increased slightly but this can be attributed to their getting older; their scores were still more externally focused than those of their nonbereaved counterparts. We also found that a low sense of self-efficacy was more common at this point when children had lost a mother. Surviving parents of children with low self-efficacy were likely to be more depressed and/or in poorer health, and to use avoidant and passive coping strategies. Because coping behavior is learned, it is not surprising that children's belief in their ability to effect change is related to the surviving parents' coping style and their parents' perceptions of their own ability to cope. In this case the surviving parents' behavior may have had a greater influence on children's self-perceptions than the loss of a parent per se.

At 1 year after the death of the parent, bereaved children who had a lower sense of self-efficacy tended to be more socially withdrawn; they had fewer friends, were less socially active, and were reluctant to talk to peers about the death of the parent. They also reported being less close to their surviving parent than children who felt more in control of events. These children also had more emotional/behavioral problems. They were likely to be depressed and anxious and reported worrying about the safety of their surviving parent. They were children who were more likely to have been told to "grow up" around the time of the death. They often came from families that experienced a significant number of concurrent losses and changes, and they themselves may have experienced a change in childcare after the parent's death.

There was no significant change in children's self-efficacy scores in the second year of bereavement, despite the fact that they were a year older. However, children with a lower sense of self-efficacy changed in other ways. They no longer showed higher levels of social withdrawal, anxiety, and depression, but instead manifested more aggressive and delinquent behavior than children who showed a more internal locus of control. They still had difficulty talking about their deceased parent and, in retrospect, felt they had not been prepared adequately for the funeral. Their relationships with their surviving parents remained poor, the latter continuing to be depressed and to adopt more passive, less effective coping strategies.

Self-Esteem

The death of a parent can affect children's self-esteem; however, this effect does not become clear until 2 years after the death. At the first anniversary of the death, the self-esteem levels of bereaved children were not significantly different from those of their nonbereaved counterparts. At the 2-year point, however, there was a large and significant difference between the self-esteem scores of the bereaved and the nonbereaved, with bereaved children reporting significantly lower self-worth. Low self-esteem was associated with more behavior problems during the first and second year of bereavement, though to a slightly lesser degree in the second year. High levels of anxiety, social withdrawal, and a lower sense of self-efficacy were also characteristic of these low-esteem children.

Maturity

We asked the children to tell us whether or not they thought they had matured because of the experience of losing a parent to death. At the 1-year point, three-quarters of the children felt more "grown up" because of this experience. Boys were more likely to feel this than girls, and more adolescents than preadolescents reported feelings of maturity. "It probably helped me mature. I am now more independent. I do more stuff, like my own school work and working around the house," said a boy who was 12 when his mother died. A girl of the same age who also lost her mother asserted, "I can take things better. After I say that I could handle my mother's death, I knew I could handle things that weren't as difficult as that." Two boys in their early teens who lost fathers expressed similar sentiments. "I feel I'm more grown up now. I've had more experiences in life and gone through more than before," said one. "I have to be, like, the man of the house, do the big chores like mow the lawn and stuff. I feel more grown up now that I'm the man of the house," reported the other. A 15-year-old boy who lost his mother had a unique perception of his maturity as he redefined the loss in his own mind and for our study: "Did you ever hear the term 'Mama's boy'? Well, now I'm not going to be one of those."

The number of children feeling grown up did not increase significantly at the 2-year anniversary of the death. However, the ratio of boys to girls with this experience had narrowed, with similar numbers of girls and boys now reporting such beliefs. By this time, more children in the study had reached adolescence, and a larger percentage of these older children reported feeling more mature than did preadolescents.

POINTS TO REMEMBER:
HOW THE CHILD RESPONDS

- Anxiety levels were higher for girls than for boys and rose significantly for all children during the first year of loss.
- Anxiety was associated with more disruption in daily life and with feeling less in control over one's circumstances.
- Crying behavior became less frequent over the 2 years of follow-up and was less frequently found in the group of adolescent boys.
- Acting-out behavior was not found with greater frequency in the bereaved group than in the matched controls. However, there was a tendency for bereaved children to show more anger at the 1-year assessment than was found in the control group.
- Somaticization and health problems were more frequent in the bereaved group, especially during the first year after death. Girls more than boys experienced these problems.
- There was an increase in accidents during the first year and this was most likely to occur in boys.
- School problems existed for some children, especially in the early months after the death, but were not more represented in the bereaved group than in the control group.

- Bereaved children, when compared to nonbereaved children, believed that they were less in control over life's circumstances both 1 and 2 years after the death.
- Changes in self-esteem began to appear 2 years after the death. At that point bereaved children rated themselves lower on these measures than did the nonbereaved children.
- Boys and adolescents were the most likely to see themselves as having matured by experiencing the death of a parent.

Mediators of the Child's Bereavement Experience

In Chapter 1 I discussed the fact that mourning is a multidetermined phenomenon. The process and outcome of bereavement is mediated by a number of factors. In Chapters 2 through 4 I described the range of children's experience. In this chapter we take a closer look at the mediating factors themselves. What specific aspects of the death, the lost parent, the surviving parent, the family, the child, and the outside world influence the course and outcome of bereavement?

THE DEATH

Type of Death

Sudden death has long been seen as more difficult to grieve than deaths in which there is some prior warning that death is imminent (Parkes, 1972). Children in the Boston study did react differently to an unexpected death. More children cried immediately after hearing the news, and fewer children attended the funeral or saw the parent's body, particularly when the children were younger. These children were less likely to feel watched by the dead parent or keep mementos of that parent. Sudden deaths also led children to have a more well-developed concept of death.

The impact of the loss was also related, to a degree, to the reaction of the surviving parent. Parents who suddenly lost their spouse reported higher levels of stress and more difficult feelings, with less opportunity to share these feelings than those parents whose spouses died expectedly. However, the results of the study show that sudden death was not associated with more emotional/behavioral difficulties on the part of the children, except at 1 year, or with any significant differences in self-esteem or feelings of self-efficacy. It is therefore likely that other factors emerged to balance the family's stress. In fact, families experiencing sudden death reported greater cohesiveness following the loss and a sense of religious and spiritual support.

Location of the Death

Where the parent dies can affect the family in different ways. When a parent died at home, children were more likely to have seen the body. In the early months after the death, these children tended to feel uneasy at the dinner table without the deceased parent. However, the study showed that location of death did not affect how frequently children talked to the dying parent, nor did it significantly affect the children's emotional/behavioral or self-perception scores following the death.

Funeral Preparation

Although emotional adjustment to loss is multidetermined, little or no preparation for the funeral was one of the strong predictors that a child would be found at risk 2 years later. Children who were not prepared for the funeral were more likely to show disturbed behavior, low self-esteem, and low self-efficacy 2 years after the death of the parent. These same children also experienced more difficulty talking about the dead parent 2 years after the loss. Those who were least likely to receive preparation tended to be younger children whose mother had died.

THE DECEASED PARENT

Gender of the Deceased

Although it is difficult to lose a parent of either gender to death, there has been speculation as to whether it is worse to lose a mother or a father. When a father dies, it is more likely that the economic status of the family will change. However, children usually lose their primary emotional caregiver with the death of a mother, as well as the stability derived from daily life routines, such as mealtimes, transportation, and being cared for when sick.

In the Child Bereavement Study it is clear that the impact of mother loss was in many ways greater than the loss of a father. Many children with mother loss suffered more emotional/behavioral problems than those with father loss. The exception was preteen boys who generally had more problems having lost a father.

Children with mother loss had lower self-esteem scores than those with father loss 2 years after the death. Children who had lost a mother also felt less in control of what was happening to them 1 year after the death.

Acting-out behavior was associated more with mother loss. For some, acting out began soon after the death and persisted at the 2-year anniversary of the loss. These findings may point to the role of the mother in limit setting, or may in some way reflect the difficulties experienced by many surviving fathers in being single parents (see Chapter 3).

The death of a mother also affected children's anxiety levels. At 1 year after the death, children with mother loss were more concerned about the safety of the surviving parent, and reported more arguments and conflict in the family and more uneasiness when coming to the diner table. This anxiety, however, attenuated during the second year of bereavement.

Although mother loss was associated with changes in sickcare, father loss was more frequently associated with the development of health problems in the early months after the death. Somaticization is a frequent expression of childhood bereavement, and becoming ill may be the child's way of obtaining reassurance from the surviving parent. One possible explanation for our finding of more illness when the mother was the surviving parent is that mothers are more likely to give hugs and tender loving care to a sick child, whereas fathers generally give medicine.

Predeath Relationship

It is no surprise that another important mediator of the course and outcome of bereavement is the predeath relationship of the child with the deceased parent. Among other things, this involves the strength of attachment, dependency issues, and, most importantly, the level of ambivalence in the relationship (Worden, 1991). Each of the above factors is influenced by the gender of the deceased parent, and the age and gender of the child him- or herself.

Families were recruited into the project after the death, so the study only provides us with a retrospective assessment of closeness from the children. The validity of retrospective data is always subject to question, especially when one is dealing with a relationship lost to death. In this context relationships are often seen as better than they might have been. With this limitation in mind, there were differences between children who saw the predeath relationship as very good and those who saw it as less good.

Those who remembered the relationship as being very good were likely to have shared interests with the dead parent, and were more likely to have stayed attached to the parent over the 2 years. Highly connected children found it easier to talk about their feelings, they cried more, and they more frequently visited the gravesite, even into the second year. They were also more likely to behave in ways that would please the dead parent.

Children with a preexisting ambivalent relationship with the deceased can be illustrated by a 15-year-old who experienced considerable anger and anxiety after the death of her stepfather. Prior to his illness their relationship was very conflicted: "He said something really mean to my sister once and I would have killed him, he got me so mad." During the stepfather's illness she did what many ambivalent people do by giving "excessive" caregiving, and she said, "I started getting along better with him." As she waited on him every morning, "I'd say do you want this or do you want that? This is the only time that we really talked." After his death she experienced considerable anger: "When I heard, I was really mad. I was nasty." She also was very fearful: "The night of the funeral, I was really scared and I was on the phone with a friend like I didn't want to go to sleep. And he [her friend] stayed up most of the night on the phone with me." By the second year she was able to resolve some of her preexisting conflicts: "I feel like I am more free now. It's not like I'm glad he's dead, but since he's died, I feel more free."

THE SURVIVING PARENT

Precisely what aspects of parental behavior influenced the course and outcome of childhood bereavement? In the Child Bereavement Study we isolated four elements of significance: the *dysfunctional* level in the surviving parent, the *discrepancy* with which the parent perceives the child, the consistency of *discipline,* and the *dating and remarriage* of the parent.

Dysfunction in the Surviving Parent

It is clear from the study that the functioning level of the surviving parent is one of the strongest mediators affecting the course and outcome of the child's bereavement. To look at the impact of dysfunction, we created a single variable that combines the parent's depression score (CES-D), the score on the IES, and the score on the Perceived Stress Scale. The most dysfunctional parents tended to be younger, had less satisfactory marriages, and did not expect their spouse to die. Many family changes (FILE) contributed to the surviving parents' stress, along with health problems, financial difficulties, and the responsibility for a larger family that included more younger children. These parents saw themselves as coping poorly, scored low on the F-COPES inventory, overused passive coping strategies, and were less skilled in reframing problems. They felt less supported than other parents in the study and found it difficult to share their feelings adequately within or outside the family.

How did this dysfunction affect the children? It consistently put the children at risk. In the early months after the death, children in these families were more withdrawn, anxious, and depressed, and experienced more sleeping difficulties. During the first and second years of bereavement these children showed more emotional/behavioral difficulties of all types, had more health problems, felt less control over events in their lives, and felt less mature than their counterparts. These children also experienced considerable social problems that persisted into the second year of bereavement. It is of interest that children with dysfunctional parents were *not* more likely to remain connected with the dead parent than those children whose parents functioned better.

Discrepancy of Perception

Another important aspect of the parent–child relationship is perceptual discrepancy—how accurately did the parent see how the child was feeling or behaving when compared to the child's report. An accurate perception is needed in order for the child to feel secure and validated. Children look to parents for validation of their own feelings, and if there is wide discrepancy, the child may feel either that the parent is "crazy" or that they themselves are "crazy." Not only does consistency in perception validate feelings for the child but it also helps the child to be able to trust his or her own feelings.

According to Winnicott (1979), a child is less anxious when the mother perceives accurately how the child is feeling. When the mother responds appropriately, the child is soothed and the anxiety level goes down. Jacobson (1954), Blanck and Blanck (1979), and other object relations theorists look at interactions with the parent as providing introjects of the parent for the child that may result in either good, positive, and soothing feelings or more unpleasant feelings such as rejection or misunderstanding. These parent–child interactions become the basis for the child's internal feeling states.

It may be difficult for bereaved parents to perceive the feelings and behavior of their children accurately for several reasons. First, the parents themselves are experiencing their own grief and may be preoccupied. Depressed parents tend to see their environment, including their children, as worse than it may be. Second, children may try to protect the parent by not revealing all that they are experiencing or feeling. Third, surviving parents take on the role of single parent and may have a need to see the child as doing better than he or she is really doing.

In the Child Bereavement Study we found that two dimensions influenced discrepancy between the parents' and the children's reports: (1) the depression of the surviving parent (the higher the depression, the greater the discrepancy) and (2) the suddenness of the death. Sudden deaths were more likely to result in discrepancy than expected deaths, with violent deaths, homicides, and suicides resulting in the highest levels of discrepancy.

How does discrepancy affect children? Two findings were

the most salient. Children who experienced higher levels of discrepancy were more likely to be anxious than were children who were perceived more accurately. Also, children experiencing discrepancy were less likely to feel in control over what was happening to them and hence expressed a more external locus of control.

Strength (1991) carried out a study of preteen children in California who had lost their fathers. She found that mothers who saw their children as being worse than the children saw themselves had children who had difficulty with anger, poor impulse control, increased anxiety, feelings of persecution, and difficulty with authority. She asked teachers to rate each child's behavior and found similar results when these independent evaluators were used. Anger control was the dimension most related to discrepancy. As in the Child Bereavement Study, Strength found that discrepancy was greater when parents were depressed and when deaths were sudden or violent.

Discipline

Limit setting can often be a problem for adults dealing with a child who has lost a parent. It is normal to feel sorry for bereaved children and to be more lenient than usual. The inability to maintain consistent disciplinary practices, combined with uncertainty as to how to respond to children's problem behavior, is frequently an issue for surviving parents.

Disciplinary problems may begin prior to the death of a parent, especially when the healthy parent is struggling with the stress of living with a terminally ill spouse. Frequently, the child's bothersome behavior stems from an increased need for attention. Some parents become restrictive and overcontrolling in an effort to achieve some impact on an environment that seems beyond their control. Restrictive discipline is also a way to cope with something concrete, namely the child's behavior.

Other parents become lax and overly indulgent. An overly permissive response may come from guilt feelings about the child's distress and the belief that tolerance can help assuage some of these guilt feelings as well as the child's pain. Overpermissiveness can also result from the parents being too depressed and withdrawn to be interested in the world around them, including the disruptive behavior of their children. Sometimes laxness reflects confusion over just what limits are appropriate for a bereaved child. A girl who moved into her teen years after the death of her mother pleaded for more consistency in discipline: "I want to have my mother around to yell at me, because I haven't been following my father's rules and teenagers need discipline." Hetherington (1979) has noted a similar lack of consistency in the application of discipline among newly separated and divorced parents; these parents also seem to make fewer demands for maturity on their children.

Strength (1991), in her study of children who had experienced father loss, found that these children functioned better when they perceived that their mothers could set more limits. Specifically, they had less difficulty with impulse control, fewer identity problems, and were less aggressive than children who perceived their mothers as being less able to set limits.

In the Child Bereavement Study we found that consistent discipline in the pre- and postdeath periods led to better outcomes for children. Poorer outcomes occurred when a mother was new to the disciplinary role; children worried more about their personal safety than those who had been disciplined by both parents before the death. When a father was new to this role, there was a greater likelihood of acting-out behavior on the part of the children. Parents may need help and encouragement from professionals working with the family to be able to evaluate and decide on appropriate and effective disciplinary strategies for bereaved children.

Dating and Remarriage

Younger parents and men were the most likely to begin dating soon after their spouse's death. In the first few months after the death, few parents (9%) in the study dated. Those who did were more likely to be men, particularly those with high levels of depression that included lower self-esteem (Worden & Silverman, 1993). These parents seemed to be reaching out for some kind of new attachment, a replacement for the lost spouse who was their primary source of support. They also had less cohesive families, were from lower socioeconomic levels, and had families who were experiencing many life-change stressors.

As the first year progressed more parents dated (37%), especially men. Children whose parents were dating during the first year experienced more emotional/behavioral problems, including somatic symptoms, withdrawn behavior, and delinquent behavior. "When my mother's boyfriend broke the TV, my brother shouted, 'My father paid for that!' It was scary," said a 9-year-old girl. "I wouldn't want him to remarry. I don't like the idea of remarriage because I don't want him to. I just don't like it. I really don't want another mother, even though I know I can't have another mother. No one else would be the same as my mother was," insisted a 12-year-old girl. She also did not want her father's girlfriend spending Christmas with them. Her 15-year-old sister held a different opinion about the woman friend: "His girlfriend is cool. If he was remarried and happy, it would be great." Also taking a more positive position on remarriage was a 10-year-old boy who said to his mother, "Are you going to get married again? I need a daddy." If a parent who was lonely began to date, it frequently made the child feel less responsible for helping the parent with the loneliness. "I think it's neat she is dating 'cause she doesn't want to be lonely for the rest of her life," reported an 11-year-old boy. Some kids pushed the dating idea. A 10-year-old girl wanted her mother to try computer dating. "She thought that you could get a fine man like him anywhere. She was just hoping," said her mother. Some children reframed the idea of remarriage by looking at their friends from divorced families: "Most of my friends have divorced parents who are going out with other people and some of them have gotten remarried again."

During the second year of bereavement, there were fewer behavioral differences between the children whose parents were dating and those who were not. Significantly, however, children of parents who were dating at this point felt more unsafe. These families also experienced a larger number of daily life changes. One girl, now 17, made this comment on her mother's dating during the second year of bereavement: "Well, sometimes I have to hide my feelings a little, just 'cause she likes going out with some guy I don't like. I know she really likes him, and I'll have to say, 'Oh, yeah, he's okay.' "

At year 2, 17% had a parent who was either engaged, living with someone, or remarried. "I felt shocked when Mom told of her plans to get married. Because it was, like, for a while we had the same old boring life. I thought it might never lighten up and then, all of a sudden, I hear she is getting married," said a 9-year-old boy. Remarriage did not seem to have an adverse effect on the children. In fact, these children experienced lower levels of anxiety and depression and were less concerned about the safety of their surviving parent than the children whose parents were not reattached. "I don't worry about her 'cause she's married and there's nothing that's going to happen to her," explained an 11-year-old girl. Remarriage was also good for the surviving parents, who reported low levels of depression, had less intrusive and avoidant thinking, and were more positive about their own coping abilities. These parents also reported lower levels of tension with their children.

THE FAMILY

How the child responds to the death of the parent is also mediated by the family and the way in which the family unit responds. All families have established working patterns that impact on the way in which the family as a unit responds to the loss. Some of the factors we will consider here include the family's size, cohesiveness, and style of coping, as well as broader variables such as family solvency and socioeconomic status.

Family Size

Family size affects the functioning of the surviving parent. Parents with a greater number of younger children at home tended to function less well, and this impacted on the children themselves. However, large families could also be a source of support for children. Children in these families reported fewer friends and more crying but also reported feeling safer. Overall, it appears that the presence of more siblings may mitigate against the influence of a poorer functioning parent and may provide children with a safe environment in which to express their feelings freely. Rosenblatt and Elde (1990) posit the need for shared reminiscences about a deceased parent and point out how siblings can fulfill this need for each other.

Family Cohesiveness

Families can be assessed on a structural continuum that ranges from "disengaged" to "enmeshed." (See FACES-III in Appendix A.) As there were only two families in the enmeshed range, most of the families in the study had scores that ranged from disengaged to connected.

Families with the highest cohesion scores tended to be headed by younger mothers. These were families where parents rated their marriage as strong and were less likely to be dating soon after the death. Cohesive families had more financial resources than those that were less engaged. Although parents in these families were stressed, they were not necessarily depressed and rated their coping as good. Their coping strategies often involved redefinition and showed an absence of passivity. Although they reported difficult feelings and having less than adequate opportunity to express these feelings, these parents had found new sources of support and derived comfort from their religious beliefs. When the death was anticipated, these were the parents who, together with their dying spouse, were most likely to plan for the future regarding finances, the funeral, and matters pertaining to the children.

Children from cohesive families showed less acting-out behavior, reported better self-esteem, and saw their conduct as better when compared to children from less cohesive families. They also reported less conflict in their families and a closer relationship with the surviving parent. Children from these families stayed connected with the dead parent through dreams and thoughts and by keeping mementos. However, they were not without difficulties. They were less likely to see the death as real and were more likely to believe that their parent was "just away" 2 years after the death. "I still keep thinking that he's going to come back in a few minutes or something," said a girl who was 10 when her father died 2 years earlier. This may relate to the fact that children in cohesive families were generally younger and the family itself in a different family stage than those families with older children. These children also had high somaticization scores that persisted 2 years after the death.

Family Stressors

Family stressors, as measured by the FILE, influenced the experience of bereavement more than any other category, both for the surviving parent and for the children. Families that have to cope with a large number of concomitant stressors occurring before and after the death are marked by increased parental stress and depression and by children with emotional/behavioral problems.

The instrument looks at 72 stressors commonly faced by families. Some of the stressors we found more frequently in the bereaved families than in the families of the control children were (1) family members with emotional problems, (2) dependence on alcohol or drugs, (3) conflict among children, (4) increased arguments between parents and children, (5) more unsolved problems, (6) chores that do not get done, and (7) increased conflict with in-laws and relatives.

Style of Coping

We found the best outcomes for both parents and children were associated with a more active coping style. Parents are frequently the models for children's coping behavior. Families who were coping the best were those who could redefine and reframe problems in a more positive way, which made these difficulties easier to deal with. Having the support of family and friends and the ability to negotiate resources in the community were also important, but to a lesser degree than active coping and reframing of problems. As shown in Chapter 6, passive coping by the surviving parent was an important risk factor for poor adjustment in the children.

Family Solvency

As might be expected, a major stressor for bereaved families is the lack of economic resources. To assess this we looked at income levels, as well as the parent's perception of the adequacy of income for the family. Although these two variables are highly correlated, there is not always a 1:1 relationship between them. Some families with less income were able to see it as adequate while the opposite was also true. Adolescents were the most sensitive about the value of money and were more concerned about having the material accoutrements to accompany their lifestyle. But overall, the lack of solvency seemed to be most important to the parents, affecting their responses to the loss more than it did for the children.

Children in families with higher incomes and more perceived solvency had higher self-esteem than children in families with lower incomes. Children from more affluent families were less likely to be in the at-risk group at any time over the 2 years. They also showed less sleep disturbance, fewer difficulties in concentration, and fewer learning problems. Income levels, however, did not affect self-efficacy—the degree to which children felt able to effect change in their lives and environment. Parents who described their finances as adequate were more likely to have done financial planning with their dying spouse, and they suffered less depression, had fewer concurrent stressors, and saw themselves as coping better.

Socioeconomic Status

Socioeconomic status is, by definition, closely related to income levels, and many of the features associated with higher income and perceived solvency are also found in families of higher socioeconomic status. However, several new features were related to families with *lower* socioeconomic status. These families were less likely to have insurance income, more likely to have parents who were dating in the early months after the death, and more likely to have rated their marriage as poorer. Their families were less cohesive and they reported less religious support. Children from these families, however, were not necessarily at more risk nor did they show poorer bereavement outcomes.

THE CHILD

Age, gender, gender match with the deceased parent, and birth order are all variables that have been shown to have an effect on the course and outcome of bereavement. In the Child Bereavement Study we identified the kinds of difficulties that were

associated with each of these factors and found that these demographics do indeed impact on the experience of loss and the child's
adaptation to the death of a parent. However, unlike other studies,
we did not find any of these variables to be so significant as actually
to predict risk status (see Chapter 6). Thus while these factors affect
the child's particular experience following the death of a parent, it
is inaccurate to make generalizations about which group of children
(older/younger, boys/girls) would find it more or less difficult to
adapt to the loss of a parent.

Age of Child

As noted earlier, the age of the child clearly has a significant impact
on the child's adaptation to the loss. Children of different ages are
grappling with different developmental tasks and the death of a
parent will almost certainly affect the way in which a child
negotiates those tasks. The Child Bereavement Study showed that
there are, indeed, several dimensions in which age affects the
bereavement experiences of children.

Preadolescence (6–11 Years)

Younger children have less well-developed cognitive and coping
skills, which means that both their emotional capacity and their
ability to understand the death will be less developed than those
of older children. We found that younger children

- Were more harassed by peers because of their parent's death.
- Experienced more social problems by the second anniversary of the death.
- Were more likely to feel watched by their deceased parent
  4 months after the death and to dream of that parent during
  the first and second years of bereavement.
- Were more likely to believe that the dead parent was "away."
- Cried more frequently.
- Had more health problems shortly after the death. For some,
  these continued into the second year when somatic symptoms were also reported in higher numbers.

Although these points indicate difficulties in adaptation, younger children often had good supports to help them. Parents with younger children reported closer and more cohesive families, more effective coping, and more access to community assistance, including both professional support and unexpected sources of support.

Adolescence (12–18 Years)

In addition to adapting to the loss, bereaved adolescents must negotiate specific developmental tasks. Fleming and Adolph (1986) have outlined three tasks that face this age group as they pass through early, middle, and later adolescence:

1. Emotional separation from their parents
2. The development of mastery and competence
3. The development of intimacy

These tasks lead the adolescent to recognize the following: "I am different from everyone else"; "I can do anything"; and "I can trust others to be there for me when needed." These tasks interface with what Fleming calls five "core issues" for the adolescent:

1. The predictability of events
2. Development of self-image
3. Belonging
4. A sense of fairness and justice
5. Mastery and control

It is Fleming and Adolph's contention that the death of a parent can affect all five of these core issues, either positively or negatively. We will return to these points at the end of this section, once we have examined how adolescents in the Child Bereavement Study were affected by the death of a parent. We compared the responses of adolescents both with preadolescents and with matched, nonbereaved adolescents in order to examine the differences between these groups.

Comparison with Preadolescents. Adolescents were more likely than preadolescents to know that their parent was going to die, and to know this for a longer period. They were more likely to attend the funeral, to be prepared for the funeral, to see the body of their dead parent, and to remember what was said at the funeral. At 2 years after the death, they were also more likely to remember the date of death. Adolescents, especially males, were the most likely to receive explicit messages from family members to act more grown up because of the loss. Although they were no more or less attached to the dead parent throughout the 2 years of follow-up, they did place more value on objects belonging to the dead parent, and kept such objects close at hand.

Bereaved adolescents had lower levels of self-esteem than bereaved preadolescents at each assessment, perhaps, in part, related to the admonition to "grow up." Unlike preadolescents, they rated their conduct as less good than their peers. However, they also reported at each assessment that they felt more mature because of the death.

Peer relationships are very important to adolescents, and they were more likely than preteens to feel like an "odd kid" because of the loss. "When people I meet ask about my mother and I tell them she died, I kinda feel different with one parent," said a 17-year-old boy. However, despite this, teens were twice as likely as preteens to talk to their friends about the dead parent.

Comparison to Nonbereaved Adolescents. During the first year following the death, bereaved adolescents were more likely to experience health problems and sleep difficulties than their matched, nonbereaved counterparts. However there were no differences in learning problems, difficulty with concentration, or in frequency of accidents. Levels of anger and delinquent behavior were also not significantly higher.

Bereaved adolescents were, however, more likely to experience tension and fighting in the family, and to report more changes at dinnertime. These differences were less significant 2 years after the death.

With regard to self-perception, bereaved adolescents saw themselves as less scholastic and less well behaved than their non-bereaved counterparts saw themselves. These differences continued into the second year. In addition, by the second anniversary of the death, bereaved adolescents reported lower self-esteem than the nonbereaved, and believed they had less control over what happened to them.

Other differences between bereaved and nonbereaved adolescents began to appear 2 years after the death. The bereaved exhibited more withdrawn behavior, had more anxiety and depression, and were more worried about how their families would function. They were also likely to be experiencing more social problems as assessed on the CBCL, though not necessarily having fewer friends.

When applying the findings from the Boston study to Fleming and Adolph's (1986) model of adolescence, we see that the death of a parent does, indeed, affect adolescents' negotiation of the core issues facing them. Concerning issue 1, the predictability of events, it is likely that the increased levels of anxiety and fear that we found among bereaved adolescents are linked to the lack of predictability in their lives caused by the death of a parent. However, levels of anger and delinquent behaviors were not significantly higher.

With regard to self-image, the second core issue, bereaved adolescents were more likely than bereaved preteens to feel like the "odd kid" and were more likely than nonbereaved adolescents to believe that their conduct and school performance were not as good as that of their peers. On the other hand, when compared to bereaved preteens, they did report that the experience had matured them. Perhaps this was compensatory behavior on their part to make up for deficits in esteem.

Bereaved adolescents showed less of a sense of belonging, the third core issue, than their nonbereaved counterparts. They had more social problems and were more withdrawn socially. We did not look at the fourth core issue, fairness and justice, but we did look at the fifth issue of mastery and control. During the second year that the effects of bereavement on mastery took their toll. It was at that point that bereaved adolescents believed they had less control over what happened to them than their nonbereaved counterparts.

Gender of Child

The impact of the child's gender on the course of mourning depends to some extent on the gender of the parent who died.

However, there were some differences when simply looking at the reactions of boys compared to girls, without reference to the gender of the dead parent. Girls, regardless of age, showed more anxiety than boys over the 2 years of bereavement. This anxiety manifested itself in concerns about the safety of the surviving parent, as well as their own safety. Girls, more than boys, were sensitive to family arguments and fights that occurred in the early months after the death.

Somatic symptoms were also more likely to be experienced by girls than boys especially 1 year after the death. Girls spoke more to their surviving parent about the death, were more likely to be crying throughout the first year of bereavement, and were more able to share feelings with the family than were boys.

Girls tended to be more attached to the dead parent than boys and, after 1 year, were more likely to idealize the deceased. At the second year assessment, they were more likely than boys to be keeping objects belonging to the dead parent close at hand.

Boys were more likely to evaluate their conduct as worse than their peers, and were more likely to have learning difficulties during the first year of bereavement. Also, boys were more likely to be given the specific dictum to "grow up" than were girls in the early months after the loss.

Gender Match

Differences in child behavior following a parent's death are related in large part to the gender of the deceased parent and, to some extent, to the gender of the child. Some children lost a parent of the same gender (match) and others a parent of the opposite gender (mismatch). All children need parental involvement, but boys and girls may look to each parent for the fulfillment of different needs (Berlinsky & Biller, 1982).

In the Child Bereavement Study we found that gender match between the child and the deceased had some impact, but to a lesser degree than we had expected. In one family where a father died, the 10-year-old daughter felt that her younger brother received more support because of gender match: "I feel that everyone gives more attention to my brother because he lost his father and I still have my mother, because he doesn't have a man. But I think

I feel the same way as him." Children who had lost a same-gender parent were more likely to identify with the dead parent and to see themselves as more like that parent than the surviving one. In the early months after the death, children who lost a same-gender parent were more likely to have objects that belonged to their parent and to keep these objects close at hand. This trend continued and more of these children reported acquiring additional objects during the second year of bereavement than did children who lost an opposite-gender parent. They also saw themselves as more mature at 1 year than did children losing opposite-gender parents.

Gender mismatch also played a part in children's bereavement experiences. Children who lost an opposite-gender parent felt more fear for the safety of the surviving parent and reported more health problems during the first year. Gender mismatch had less influence during the second year of bereavement.

The differences described above apply to both boys and girls. There was one significant set of differences that applied only to girls. Girls who experienced mother loss had more emotional/behavioral problems at the first year assessment. Of particular note was the high delinquent score at both 4 months and 1 year. Not only did the fathers rate the conduct of these girls as bad, but the girls themselves rated their own conduct as less good than their peers. This acting-out behavior attenuated during the second year of loss, and at the second year assessment many of these same girls reported acting good to please the dead parent.

It may be that gender-match effects will be seen later as the children move into young adulthood. Learning of sex roles is an important aspect of children's development and persons other than parents can serve as such role models. There is some evidence from other studies, however, that females who have lost a father during childhood have different relationships with males than those not bereaved (Berlinsky & Biller, 1982; Hetherington, 1972).

Birth Order

Studies of birth order show that first-borns are highly oriented toward parents in terms of standards of conduct and sensitivity to evaluation by the parent. We wanted to see what, if any, bereavement effects could be seen when first-borns were compared with children born second or later. For purposes of this analysis, we excluded single-child families and controlled for age, because first-borns tended to be older.

We found that first-borns were more likely to know about a pending death for a longer period of time. During the early months following the death, the first-borns saw themselves as more like the dead parent than the surviving parent, when compared to children born later. They were also more likely to keep objects belonging to the deceased, and this continued into the second year of bereavement. Anxiety was high amongst first-borns, with more concern about personal safety and more uneasiness at the dinner table. During the first and second years of bereavement, first-born children were sensitive to and noted changes in the surviving parent. They also behaved in ways that would please the dead parent.

Understanding of Death

The impact of death on children depends in part on their understanding of death. As discussed in Chapter 1, very young children do not have the mental capacity to understand abstractions such as finality and irreversibility. They may, in fact, see death as reversible, as the following incident illustrates: A friend of mine buried the family dog in the backyard garden; her son, age 3 at the time, thought the dog would come up in the spring along with the tulips they had planted. As children grow older, they develop the capacity to understand the abstractions associated with death.

In the Child Bereavement Study we monitored children's understanding of death in the 2 years following the loss of the parent. Clearly, one would expect some changes as the children got older and their cognitive capacities matured. However, we wanted to see whether children who have experienced death first hand would have more well-developed concepts of death than children who had not had such experiences.

Both the bereaved children and their matched, nonbereaved counterparts were assessed in terms of the ability to understand death, including four concepts associated with a mature under-standing of death, namely, irreversibility, finality, inevitability, and causality (Smilanski, 1987). Contrary to our expectations, non-bereaved children had more well-developed concepts of death than bereaved children at both the first and second year assess-ments. Of the four concepts, causality and finality were most pronounced in favor of the control children. Bereaved children's understanding of three of these four categories matured in the 2 years following the death; however, there was no significant maturing of their concept of causality. During the first year of bereavement there was a decided maturing of the concept of finality, in particular, as children grappled with the reality of the loss. However, this concept was still less developed for bereaved children than for their nonbereaved counterparts. One wonders if bereaved children would not allow themselves to believe in finality to the fullest extent because they were struggling to relocate the deceased parent in their lives.

There was no significant change in bereaved children's total understanding of death scores between the first and second year assessments. Neither the gender of the lost parent nor that of the child were significantly correlated with an understanding of death. Surprisingly, there was no simple correlation between an under-standing of death and the child's age; some older children had less developed concepts while some younger children had a very mature understanding of death.

If age and gender were not significant correlates, what were? Children with a more mature understanding of death in the early months were those who had attended the funeral and who had gone to the gravesite at some point during the first year. Sudden or violent deaths, such as by accident, suicide, or homicide, were also associated with a more mature understanding. When the death was expected, children who had talked about death with their dying parent were also likely to have more mature concepts.

A higher level of death understanding did affect behavior in the first year. Early on, these children had more social problems, anxiety, depression, and aggression than did children with less mature concepts of death. However, these behaviors were also associated with parent vulnerability and that influence must be taken into consideration.

POINTS TO REMEMBER:
MEDIATORS OF THE CHILD'S
BEREAVEMENT EXPERIENCE

- Losing a parent suddenly leads to a worse adaptation to loss at 1 year. It does not lead to lower self-esteem or to less belief in one's ability to control one's environment.
- Having a parent die at home neither increases communication between the children and the dying parent nor portends a better or worse adjustment afterwards.
- In general, the loss of a mother is worse for most children than the loss of a father. This is especially true as one moves through the second year of bereavement. The death of a mother portends more daily life changes and, for most families, the loss of the emotional caretaker for the family.
- Mother loss is associated with more emotional/behavioral problems including higher levels of anxiety, more acting-out behavior, lower self-esteem, and less belief in self-efficacy.
- Mother loss brings about more connection with the dead parent.
- The functioning level of the surviving parent is the most powerful predictor of a child's adjustment to the death of a parent. Children with a less well-functioning parent will show more anxiety and depression, and sleep and health problems.
- Bereaved children will have fewer emotional/behavioral problems if discipline is consistently administered and if the surviving parent perceives the child's needs and behavior in a way that is similar to the child's perception. Inconsistent discipline and perceptual discrepancies will lead to high levels of anxiety in the child.
- Parental dating in the first year of bereavement can be associated with significant problems in the children including withdrawn behavior, acting-out behavior, and somatic symptoms. This was especially true when the surviving parent was a father.
- The effects of engagement or remarriage after a suitable bereavement period, on the other hand, can be positive, with children in these families experiencing lower levels of anxiety and depression as well as being less concerned about the safety of the surviving parent.

• Having a number of siblings can have a positive effect in child bereavement. This can mitigate against the negative effects of having a less well-functioning parent. Also, larger families provide a context of safety that gives a child the opportunity and encouragement to express feelings.

• Cohesive families will have children who show less acting-out behavior and who feel better about themselves than children who come from less cohesive families.

• Families that experience large numbers of concomitant stressors occurring before and after the death will have parents with more stress and depression and children who show more emotional/behavioral problems.

• The best bereavement outcomes occur in families who cope actively rather than passively and in families who can find something positive in a difficult situation.

• Bereaved children did not have more well-developed understandings of death than did control children, despite having experienced the death of a parent.

S · I · X

Children at Risk

Are parentally bereaved children more at risk for high levels of emotional/behavioral difficulties than nonbereaved children? If so, when is this risk the highest? In this chapter I will try to answer these questions. In the Child Bereavement Study we first compared bereaved children with their nonbereaved counterparts to assess just how significant the differences in risk frequencies between them were. We also assessed what factors might predict future risk, or which grief reactions—or combination of reactions—facilitate adjustment to loss. Finally, I look beyond our study to review the literature dealing with long-term consequences of parental death during childhood.

To define at-risk behavior, we used scores from the CBCL. Children whose scores on this inventory of emotional/behavioral problems exceeded 64 were placed in the risk group for that time point (i.e., time of assessment—4 months, 1 year, 2 years). This T-score value of 64 is the criterion level established by the test author (Achenbach, 1991) to discriminate between children whose problems warrant referral to mental health resources from those whose problems do not.

BEREAVEMENT AND RISK: A "LATE EFFECT"?

In order to assess differences between bereaved and nonbereaved children, we compared the risk percentages of the children in the Child Bereavement Study with those of their matched nonbereaved counterparts. At 1 year after the death, 19% of the bereaved children fell into the at-risk group, compared to only 10% of the nonbereaved children. Although there was a larger percentage of bereaved children at risk, this difference only approached statistical significance. However, 2 years after the death, there were significantly more bereaved than nonbereaved children in the risk group (21% as compared to 6% of the nonbereaved). This large and significant difference was one of the most important findings from the study. It suggests that there is a "late effect" of bereavement for a significant minority of these school-age children, and emphasizes the importance of regular follow-up assessments of children over a longer period of time.[1]

To measure just how large this late effect might be, we calculated the "attributable risk percentage" (G. W. Brown & Harris, 1986) both 1 and 2 years after the death. This figure identifies the percentage of emotional disturbance that can be attributed to the crises event (the death) and its consequences within the family. Our results showed that the attributable risk percentage doubled from Year 1 (35%) to Year 2 (75%), further indicating the existence of a "late effect" phenomenon by which more of the serious emotional/behavioral problems at 2 years could be attributed to the experience of losing a parent to death. This finding makes a strong case for the identification of children who will be at risk 1 and 2 years after the death so that early intervention to can take place to preclude this late effect. (A screening instrument for the early identification of children at risk was developed using the data from the Child Bereavement Study. See Chapter 9 and Appendix B for details.)

RISK PREDICTORS

In Chapter 5 we identified factors that influence the course and outcome of bereavement. Now let us examine just how these factors interact and play out in the lives of bereaved children and how they correlate with risk membership (i.e., inclusion in the at-risk category) at each assessment (see also Table 1). The results of this study highlight the strong predictive weight of the family context and, most particularly, the functioning of the surviving

---

[1]Overall, a total of 36% of the children fell into the at-risk group at one or more of the assessement points.

TABLE 1. Determinants of Risk Membership by Time

	4 months	1 year	2 years
Death and rituals			
Sudden death	−	+	−
Violent death	−	+	−
No funeral preparations	−	+	+
Not expect death	+	+	−
The deceased parent			
Can't speak of parent	+	−	−
Idealizes deceased	+	−	+
Guilt/regrets	+	−	+
High levels of grief	−	+	−
Uneasy at dinner table	−	+	×
Understanding of death	+	+	−
The surviving parent			
Perceived stress	+	+	+
Depressed	+	+	−
Intrusive thoughts	−	+	+
Not employed	+	−	+
Avoidant thinking	−	+	−
Passive coping style	+	+	+
Perceived poor coping	−	+	−
Health problems	+	−	−
New losses	×	×	+
Less prepared for death	+	+	−
Connected to spouse	×	+	−
Lacking support	×	+	+
Change in routine	−	+	+
The family			
More family stressors	+	+	+
More younger children	+	−	−
Tension and arguments	−	+	+
Unhelpful in-laws	−	−	+
The child			
Age of child	−	−	−
Gender of child	−	−	−
Gender match	−	−	−
Low self-esteem	+	+	−
Low self-efficacy	+	+	+
Feels unsafe	−	+	−
Fears parent safety	−	−	+
Less peer support	+	−	−

Note. + = risk determinant; − = not a risk determinant; × = not assessed.

parent in the adjustment of children. Such factors can impact in either positive or negative ways, depending on how well or how badly the individual parent is coping.

Unlike some other studies that report specific high-risk groups such as teenage boys who lose their fathers or preschoolers who lose their mothers (Berlinsky & Biller, 1982; Osterweis et al., 1984), we did not find the demographics of the child (age, gender, and gender match) alone to be significant predictors of risk status. Some of these previous studies were based on less adequate data and often failed to take into account specific family data such as the functioning of the surviving parent or the adequacy of parenting after the death.

In the following section one can see which factors contributed to risk at each assessment point. The most salient predictors are listed first, with other contributing variables mentioned afterward. As time progressed, some factors continued to be important risk factors. However, significant new factors also emerged at each assessment point.

Four Months

At 4 months after the death, children at risk could be most clearly identified by the following discriminating factors:

- Lower self-esteem
- More difficulty speaking about the dead parent
- Expected death for a briefer period of time
- More likely to have experienced some type of accident during this period

Other factors distinguishing these children from those not at-risk at this point include a lower sense of self-efficacy; difficulties with peers and a lack of peer support; and more understanding of the finality of death.

The most salient *family influences* that discriminated at-risk children from those not at risk in these early months include the following:

- Many family stressors and changes
- Less time for the surviving parent to prepare for the death

- A parent experiencing health problems and/or depression
- Passive coping style

Other family factors contributing to risk membership at this point include a surviving parent not being employed or not having a salary income, a parent experiencing high levels of stress and coping less well, and a larger number of younger children in the family.

First Year

At 1 year after the death, children at high risk were most characterized by the following:

- Feelings of anxiety, most particularly concerning personal safety and uneasiness at the dinner table
- Lower self-esteem
- Experiencing a sudden or violent death
- Little or no preparation for the funeral

At-risk children also felt less good about themselves and believed they had less control over events in their lives (low self-efficacy). They reported more tension in the family and felt less close to their surviving parent. In addition to the feelings of anxiety mentioned above, at-risk children experienced more headaches and difficulties in concentration. Also, they remembered their dead parents with considerable sadness.

Factors affecting the family as a whole included the following:

- The suddenness of the death
- The number of family stressors and changes
- The fact that the surviving parent made little or no effort to dispose of personal belongings of the deceased

At the first anniversary, parents of at-risk children reported more tension with the children. They continued to report more stresses and changes in family life and routine, with high levels of depression, stress, and intrusive thoughts of the deceased. They perceived themselves as coping poorly and continued to have passive coping styles. These highly distressed parents also reported less support from family and friends. One can speculate that children at risk at this time, who were likely to have a more mature understanding of the finality of death, may have been confused by the continuing presence of the belongings of the dead parent in the household. As shown above, suddenness of death, especially when the death was violent (accident, suicide, homicide), became an important discriminator between high and low risk at this time.

Second Year

At 2 years after the death, the strongest predictors of risk at this time were that children had experienced:

- Little or no preparation for the funeral
- Fear about the safety of the surviving parent

During this period, low self-esteem was no longer a significant correlate of grief, while lower self-efficacy continued to be an important predictor. As mentioned earlier, this may be related to the fact that coping behavior is learned and surviving parents still modeled less effective coping. These children were more likely to idealize the dead parent. They reported higher levels of grief and sadness and felt some responsibility for the death. At-risk children were not able to redesign the funeral of their lost parent. As mentioned above, these were children who were given little or no preparation for the funeral.

The most salient parent and family predictors at this time were as follows:

- High levels of family stressors and change
- Many changes in the parent's routine
- Less helpful in-laws
- Parent's passive coping style

Parents continued to feel high levels of stress, with escalating tensions and clashes with children, many of whom were moving into adolescence. Other stressors included continuing health problems, additional losses, and new problems with which to cope. Support from family and friends seemed to be lacking, with parents feeling that their needs were not being met. Levels of grief were high for these parents, who often pushed themselves to "get over it."

RISK PROFILES

Once a child is at risk, does he or she continue to be at risk over the following 2 years? The answer is no. In the study there were children (10%) who did fall into the risk category at each assessment. There were others (12%), however, who fell into the risk group shortly after the death but were not at risk 1 and 2 years later. There were still others (14%) who were not at risk early on, but did fall into the risk group either at 1 or 2 years. And, there was, of course, a large group of children (65%) who never fell into the risk group at any time during the 2 years of follow-up. I want to contrast the profiles of children at continued risk and those who were never at risk.

Continued Risk

There were several factors that put children at continued risk, among them the loss of a parent by sudden or violent death. These children had a more well-developed concept of death early on and did not feel watched by their dead parent. Early in the mourning process they experienced more health problems and accidents. During the first year of loss they reported feeling increasingly sad and they felt closer to the dead parent than they did to the living parent. During the second year they felt some blame regarding the loss and experienced learning difficulties.

Families of these continued risk children experienced higher levels of concurrent stressors, including financial difficulties; they coped using passive coping styles; and they generally felt less supported by others, including in-laws and extended family. Age, gender, gender of the lost parent, and gender match did not distinguish membership in the continued risk group.

Never at Risk

There were 81 children who never fell into the risk group at any time during the 2 years of follow-up. Not only were their behavior scores in the normal ranges but the children themselves reported fewer health and sleep disturbance problems 4 months after the death. They were socially active and had a sense of self-efficacy, believing that they could have some influence over what was happening to them. It is possible that some of these children may not have adequately grappled with the reality of their parent's death. At the first assessment, these no-risk children had a less mature understanding of the finality and causality of death. They also were less likely to have revisited the gravesite.

During the first year of bereavement, the no-risk children experienced significantly fewer changes and disruptions in their daily lives than children at risk. They reported feeling safer and more in control of their lives, had fewer concentration and learning problems, and experienced fewer health problems and somatic complaints. They were no more nor less connected to the dead parent; were more likely to believe that their parent was in a specific place, such as heaven; and were unlikely to feel any responsibility for the death.

During the second year, these no-risk children continued to feel more in control over their circumstances. They were less fearful regarding the safety of their surviving parent, were not feeling blame for the death, and reported being a good child for the benefit of their dead parent. These children also were more likely to have been prepared by adults for the funeral, and when asked at 2 years if they would like to come up with a revised funeral for the dead parent, they were more likely to do this.

The no-risk children had surviving parents who were slightly older, and they came from families with fewer younger children. Over the 2 years, these surviving parents reported less stress, depression, and intrusive thoughts of the deceased. The families experienced fewer concurrent stressors and fewer changes in daily family life. When faced with difficulties, these surviving parents coped by using active coping strategies more often than passive ones. Parents of no-risk children reported fewer health problems, felt like their support was adequate, and were less likely to seek out professional support. They also reported less tension with their children than parents whose children fell into the higher risk groups.

LONG-TERM CONSEQUENCES

Findings from the Child Bereavement Study have shown the short-term consequences (first 2 years) of parental death on school-age children, but what are the long-term consequences (when children reach adulthood) of such a loss? There has been a longstanding interest in this question, beginning with Freud in his classic paper *Mourning and Melancholia* (1917). Freud posited that an incomplete mourning as a child would make one vulnerable to adult depression.

Many clinicians and researchers have gone on to examine a variety of symptoms and behaviors in an attempt to establish a relationship between childhood loss and adult health and mental health outcomes. (There has also been a similar interest in adult outcomes for children of divorced families; see, e.g., Wallerstein, 1991.) The results of these studies are conflicting, but it is clear that not all children who experience parental loss go on to develop adult psychopathology. There are still many questions regarding why it is that some individuals are resilient while others are vulnerable and go on to develop long-term problems. Most of the investigations of long-term consequences focus on psychological, medical, and behavioral consequences of childhood parental loss. In this section we will look at some of the findings in these areas, as well as the limitations of the research to date.

Psychological Consequences

Depression

Following Freud's lead, the most frequently studied long-term consequence of early parental loss has been depression (Barnes & Prosen, 1985; Finkelstein, 1988; Klerman & Weissman, 1986; Tennant et al., 1980, 1981; Wilson et al., 1967). The assumption underlying this possible relationship is the idea that losses in adulthood reactivate the trauma associated with childhood loss. Research data linking early loss and adult depression are often conflicting and only suggestive. Lloyd (1980) examined 11 studies and found that in 8 of the 11 there was a link between childhood bereavement and adult depression. It appears that childhood loss of a parent increased the risk of depression by a factor of 2 to 3. Lloyd also noted that early loss correlated with the severity of the depression.

In Britain G. W. Brown and colleagues (1977) compared a

group of depressed women with a group of matched nondepressed controls. Women in the depressed group had a higher incidence of maternal death before age 11.

However, data on this relationship are not consistent across studies. Others, such as Tennant et al. (1980), have urged caution about positing such a relationship. Additional factors, such as the quality of relationship with a subsequent caretaker, may be more influential in determining the risk for later depression than simply the experience of bereavement itself (Birtchnell, 1980).

Suicide

Depression is frequently a factor in suicidal behavior and there have been studies that looked for a relationship between childhood bereavement and adult suicidal behavior (Birtchnell, 1970b; Crook & Raskin, 1975; Dorpat et al., 1965; Farberow et al., 1987; Goldney, 1981; Hill, 1969; Levi et al., 1966). In one study Birtchnell (1972) found that twice as many depressed suicide attempters were parentally bereaved compared with nonsuicidal depressives. However, studies looking at this phenomenon have not been consistent and the confounding effects between depression and suicidal behavior have often contributed to this inconsistency.

Anxiety Disorders

A more recent area of investigation for the long-term consequences of childhood bereavement has been that of anxiety disorders (Coryell et al., 1983; Faravelli et al., 1985; Raskin et al., 1982; Tennant et al., 1980; Torgersen, 1986; Tweed et al., 1989). These studies have suggested that there is a relationship between premature parental loss and the development of anxiety disorders.

A recent and well-done study looked at the incidence of adult psychopathology in a large group of female twins who had been separated from a parent prior to age 17 (Kendler et al., 1992). One-third of the losses were due to death and two-thirds due to separations from other causes. They found that increased risk for generalized anxiety disorder was associated with parental separation but not with parental death. However, the risk for a diagnosis of panic disorder did turn out to be associated with parental loss by death, as was the risk for the diagnosis of phobia. Of interest is the fact that this study did not find a significant relationship between parental death and adult depression, thus the study argues against the earlier conclusion of Tennant and colleagues (1980) that the impact of loss is greater on depression than on anxiety states.

Psychoses

There was an attempt in the 1960s and 1970s to find a relationship between childhood bereavement and the risk of developing schizophrenia. Dennehy (1966), Oltman and Friedman (1965), and Watt and Nicholi (1979) reported such an association between early parental death and schizophrenia. However, others have found no supportive evidence for such an association (Birtchnell, 1972; Granville-Grossman, 1966). More recent research has identified biological and genetic parameters of schizophrenia and the interest in childhood bereavement and schizophrenia has waned.

Medical Consequences

As in the case for psychological consequences, the evidence that childhood bereavement affects health status as an adult is mixed. Several studies have suggested that children losing a parent to death are more likely to demonstrate symptomatology, to have increased utilization of healthcare resources, and to demonstrate more complaints of ill health in adult life (Raphael, 1983; Seligman et al., 1974). Supporting this is the study of Bendiksen and Fulton (1975). They followed prospectively a group of ninth-graders into their 30s and found that children with earlier loss were more susceptible to serious medical illnesses than were the control subjects in their study. However, the exact nature of these illnesses was not specified by the authors.

Behavior Disorders

A third area that has been investigated as a long-term consequence of childhood bereavement has been that of antisocial personality (F. Brown & Epps, 1966; Markusen & Fulton, 1971; Rutter, 1984). Again, the findings have been mixed and inconclusive. Markusen and Fulton (1971) found that men who were bereaved in childhood were more likely to be law breakers when in their 20s than were nonbereaved men in the control group. F. Brown and Epps (1966) studied a group of prisoners consisting of both men and women. They found an excess of parental death in this group of prisoners.

Reasons for Inconclusive Findings

There are several reasons as to why the information on the long-term impact of parental loss is inconsistent and inconclusive. First, most of the studies have been retrospective. They identify a target group such as depression or criminality and then try to measure the frequency of parental loss in that target group as compared to a control group. A prospective study in which children would be followed over time would not only help to identify long-term risk frequency but would also help to identify factors that lead to risk in some children and to resiliency in others.

A lack of attention to confounding variables is a second limitation of most long-term consequence studies. Variables that need to be accounted for include the age of the child at the time of loss, gender of the deceased parent, the cause of death, the quality of relationship with deceased and surviving parents, and the kind of parenting the child received after the loss.

A third limitation of some studies is the tendency to lump together all types of parental loss whether by death, divorce, or some other reason for abandonment (Breier et al., 1988; T. Harris et al., 1986; Tennant, 1988). The impact of these different losses may play out in various ways, and it is important to sort out impact by type of loss. A few studies have done this and found significant qualitative differences depending on the type of loss (Kendler et al., 1992).

Sampling weaknesses are the fourth reason for these inconclusive findings. Some of the reports have been based on patient samples, others have been based on case studies or clinical observations (Bowlby, 1960), while still others have samples that are of inadequate size. Associated with sampling problems is the lack in many of these studies of appropriate controls.

A fifth reason for discrepancies is the lack of adequate theory to undergird these findings. There has been little attention given to determining the processes by which early loss leads to the development of psychopathology in adulthood. Not all children who experience parental loss go on to develop adult psychopathology, and the factors that predict the development of such conditions following early loss have not been determined. Important factors that may contribute to the development of psychopathology following loss, such as genetic predisposition to disorders or the effects of loss on long-term neurobiological functioning, have been overlooked (Breier et al., 1988). The few existing theories include the following:

- Psychodynamic theory has been used to identify possible precursors of later pathology. The loss of a parent with whom the child has an insecure attachment and the failure of the child to internalize the deceased parent are posited as major contributors to later psychopathology (Bowlby, 1982; Vaillant, 1985).
- Another theory suggests that outcomes of parental loss are related to "perceived vulnerability." People who experience negative life events perceive themselves as being more vulnerable to these types of experiences than do others without the same history (Perloff & Fetzer, 1986). Mireault and Bond (1992) studied a group of college students who experienced parental death in childhood to see whether they were more likely to perceive themselves and significant others to be more vulnerable to death than people who have not had this type of loss experience. They found that this group perceived themselves as more vulnerable to future loss than a nonbereaved control group. This perceived vulnerability to loss was a better predictor of adult anxiety and depression than was the earlier loss taken alone. Mireault and Bond caution that the clinician or researcher should not assume that an adult client's anxiety or depression is linked simply and directly to grief over an early loss without considering the cognitive factor of perceived vulnerability.

Some Recent Directions

I was recently invited to be a discussant on a national television program, where the topic for the day was mother loss. Several adults were invited to share their experience and to discuss how the loss of a mother during childhood had affected their adult life. Each of the participants spoke about the ongoing influence of such a loss and of the need to rethink who that parent would have been in their current life, had the parent survived. This ongoing review of how the relationship might have been is similar to the experiences reported by Wellesley women students interviewed by Silverman (1989). After the program I received a number of calls from people looking for a support group including others who had lost a parent. Finding out that others also had their lingering questions and longings gave these callers impetus to share their experience. The book by Hope Edelman (1994) on motherless daughters has been a recent bestseller in which women of different ages speak of the ongoing impact of mother loss on their present lives. These women articulated what they were missing by not having a mother at various life cycle stages. There also are books that examine the ongoing impact of father loss (M. Harris, 1995).

It may be that the most important long-term consequence of parental death during childhood is neither depression nor anxiety disorder, as important as these are, because these only affect a small percentage of adults with childhood parental loss. Rather, the most important long-term impact may be their continuing sense of emptiness and an ongoing need to rethink who this parent would have been in their lives had he or she remained alive. This ongoing presence of the lost parent is strong for most people, even though they may have had adequate parenting by the surviving parent or parent surrogate.

POINTS TO REMEMBER:
CHILDREN AT RISK

- At 1 and 2 years after the death of a parent, the percentage of bereaved children in the high-risk group exceeds that for matched nonbereaved control children. This difference is greater at 2 years than at 1 year.
- The percentage of risk attributable to the death of a parent doubles from Year 1 to Year 2, arguing for a late effect of the loss on these children.

- Consistent family risk predictors over the 2 years included a larger number of younger children in the home, higher levels of concurrent family stressors, inadequate support from family and others, and passive coping styles of the surviving parent.
- Consistent child risk predictors included low self-efficacy, fear for surviving parent's safety, idealizing the deceased parent, poor social relationships, and higher levels of grief and sadness.
- Child demographic factors such as gender, age, and gender match with the deceased parent did not contribute to risk as significantly as might be expected.
- Although a third of the bereaved children experienced serious emotional/behavioral difficulties at some point during the first 2 years after the loss, two-thirds of the children did not experience such difficulties.
- Evidence for long-term consequences for parentally bereaved children is inconclusive. There is more evidence for depression risk and panic attacks, and less for generalized anxiety disorders, suicide, and conduct disorders.
- Ongoing meaning making for adults who lost parents as children involves not only why their parent left them but also who this parent would now be in their adult lives.

COMPARATIVE LOSSES

When a Sibling Dies

When considering childhood bereavement, the question arises as to how children's responses to the death of a parent may differ from their responses to the death of a sibling? Is the course and outcome of mourning similar or different? What issues need to be negotiated by children who lose a parent, and how do these compare to those facing children who lose a sibling?

DISTINGUISHING FEATURES
OF SIBLING LOSS

I have identified 13 features that differentiate sibling loss from parental loss. These features provide insight as to how and why the course of bereavement may be affected by these two different types of family loss.

Impact of the Loss on Parents

The impact of any loss is multidetermined, and this makes it difficult to compare one type of loss with another. Nevertheless, some believe that the loss of one's child, especially when the child is a minor, is among life's most devastating. Sanders (1979–1980) compared groups of people who had sustained the loss of a child, a spouse, or a sibling and found that those respondents who had lost a child had some of the highest grief scores, even years after the death.

Children who lose a parent to death, as well as those who lose a sibling, will be faced with grieving parents whose own grief may make it difficult for them to be emotionally available or to parent effectively. However, those children who have a sibling die may have parents who are experiencing more intense levels of grief and for whom the grief continues for a longer time period than children who have a parent die (Rosen, 1985).

Availability of One Parent versus Two

The child whose mother or father dies is faced with a single-parent family and all that entails. We have already looked at the notion that bereaved children who lose a sibling are faced with the unavailability of one or both parents because of the parents' grief. However, it is always possible that one parent's grief may be less intense than the other's and that this parent may be more available to recognize and respond to the needs of the children. In the case of the single parent, the child is dependent on the functioning of that one person. In either situation adults other than the parents can help the children during the days and months following the death. Sociologist Robert Fulton (personal communication, 1995) calls these adults "intimate strangers" and points out their importance in the life and functioning of a bereaved child.

Tensions in the Marriage

Marital tensions after the death often occur in sibling loss, with statistics differing as to the divorce potential following the death of a child. Whatever the percentages are, investigators seem to agree, however, that parents who divorce after a child's death often have preexisting tensions in the marriage (Worden & Monahan, 1993). The death of the child serves to increase marital tension and provides the couple with the opportunity to separate. Whatever the actual percentage of divorce among bereaved parents, the sickness and death of a child can create an imbalance in a couple's relationship, bringing some couples closer together and causing others to move apart. This possibility of marital tension after the death is unique to the loss of a sibling and would, of course, not be present for children who lost a parent to death.

Increased "Personal Death Awareness"

"Personal Death Awareness" (Worden, 1976) refers to one's awareness of one's own mortality—an awareness we all have at a low
level most of the time. This awareness becomes more figural when
we are confronted by a near accident, the death of a contemporary,
a serious illness, or other potential losses. Children who lose a
sibling experience a higher increase in personal death awareness
than those who lose a parent (Rosen & Cohen, 1981). When a
sibling dies, the child must confront the fact that he or she could
also die, something known to a greater or lesser degree depending
on age, but something that is hardly ever a focus in the child's daily
existence.

Personal death awareness often brings with it an increased
concentration of anxiety, especially existential anxiety, which can
manifest itself in a child's life in a number of ways. Some children
become phobic concerning certain items or circumstances, including fear of leaving the primary attachment figure—the surviving
parent. For other children, anxiety can be manifested through
somatic symptoms. In still other cases the anxiety may be chal-
lenged through risk-taking behavior, with the child trying to show
fearlessness or invincibility by successfully accomplishing certain
high-risk activities.

Replacing the Lost Sibling

Bereaved parents may subtly or otherwise push another child to
replace the lost sibling. What is being replaced depends on the
roles that the deceased child played in the family, including gender
roles (Cain et al., 1964). For example, one family had several
daughters before a son was born. He died when he was 6 and his
father was devastated to lose his only son. Over the years the father
encouraged the daughter who was closest in age to the deceased
to participate in activities usually reserved for fathers and sons. This
girl gradually developed certain masculine interests that may not
have developed if her brother had lived.

Not only do parents look to other children to help make up
for a child's loss, children may place pressure on themselves to do
this. They see the devastation the death has caused their parents

and they want to do something to ease the pain and to make things better (Hogan, 1988). In one family the child who died was an accomplished athlete, something his father aspired to but never achieved. After the boy was killed in an accident, the brother attempted to take up the sport in which the deceased had excelled. This was very awkward for the brother, who tried for many months but was unsuccessful in the sport because he did not possess his sibling's natural athletic abilities.

Overprotecting the Surviving Children

Although it is possible that a parent whose spouse dies will be protective of the children, it is more likely that parents who lose a child will be overprotective of the remaining children. Krell and Rabkin (1979) point this out as one of the common results of parental bereavement. To protect one's children is a normal part of the role of a parent. A child's death causes parents to confront their inability to protect the child and this adds to the stress of the loss. Overprotection of the surviving children can be a counter to this stress. Although this may make the parent feel better, such overprotection can thwart a child's development, particularly at the point of autonomy and individuation. The child whose parent dies is less likely to be the recipient of such overprotection.

Focus of Blame and Scapegoating

When confronted with the death of a loved one, many people need to blame someone or something for the loss (Tooley, 1975). The need to blame is especially common when the loss is violent, as in the case of a homicide or suicide, as well as with certain accidental deaths. Blame can be assigned within as well as outside the family. In some bereaved families a surviving child is the most convenient target for scapegoating. Siblings of a dead child can become the targets of such accusations, with parents or other family members blaming a child for contributing to the death through some action taken or not taken. If a parent feels responsible for the death of a child, he or she may not be able to cope with the intensity of the guilt, which then may be projected onto another family member, often a child. Such projected blame could happen after the death of a parent, but we saw very little of this in the Child Bereavement Study. Only eight children reported such behavior in their families. In my clinical experience I have seen more scapegoating behavior in families where a child died than in families where a parent died.

Jealousy of the Sick Sibling

Although accidents are a major cause of child deaths, many children also die of illnesses, often lengthy and with many hospitalizations. When this is the case, a parent is often preoccupied with the welfare of the sick child and with the care of this child. Such appropriate concern can be a source of conflict for the other children in the family, who see the parents' attention to their ill sibling as a point of neglect of themselves. These children may come to resent the sick child for getting all of the attention. After the sibling dies, this resentment can cause conflicts for the remaining children and lead to feelings of guilt and anger, frequently the results of a preexisting ambivalent relationship with the sibling who died (Krell & Rabkin, 1979).

Survivor Guilt

Survivor guilt is often experienced by the people who remain alive after a loved one dies. Such guilt is frequently found when two people experience the same disaster or tragedy and one dies while the other survives. Survivor guilt can be especially strong when many people die, as in the case of a natural disaster, and only a few survive. Survivors are confronted with the question, "Why me?" Some move forward with their lives and find a purpose to survivorship, while others remain plagued with a sense of guilt and uneasiness (Fanos & Nickerson, 1991).

Children who lose a sibling may experience this type of guilt: "Why was my brother killed and not me?" Such survival guilt, though not common, is more likely to be a feature of sibling loss than of parental death.

Anger at Parents for Not Protecting the Sibling

Earlier I discussed the role of the parent as protector until the children are able to care for themselves. Some bereaved children feel an uneasiness and resentment that their parents were not able to protect their sibling from death (Rosen & Cohen, 1981). This is more likely the case in an accidental or violent death than in a natural death, but even when death is from natural causes anger still can occur. For most children this is not necessarily a conscious response, but one that may reside more on the preconscious level and underlie some of the acting-out behavior seen in children after the death of a sibling. In rare cases children will become highly independent, wanting to care for themselves, excessively taking care of other people, and not wanting to be dependent on others.

Residue of Sibling Competition

Although it is possible for children to compete with a parent, such competitiveness bears little resemblance to the competitive relationships many siblings have with each other. If the sibling competitor dies, the surviving sibling may experience a sense of relief, which is usually short lived and which often turns into feelings of guilt that one remains or has won at the expense of the other. It is important that children be allowed to talk about these feelings with someone who will understand and not be judgmental.

The Wrong Child Died

Another possible consequence of sibling death is the feeling on the part of a parent that the wrong child died. Some parents may directly articulate this to a child: "You should have died and not your sister." Other parents holding such a feeling will not necessarily be so explicit, but this unarticulated feeling will be in the background and will most certainly affect the child's life as well as the child's relationship with that parent.

One family lost their 14-year-old son when he was riding in a car with a 16-year-old friend who had just gotten his driver's license. The whole family was devastated by this tragedy, but it was especially hard for the father, who had a close relationship with the boy. In this family there were two surviving siblings, a brother and a sister. The father wished that his 17-year-old son had been the one to die and not the younger one, but he did not voice this thought to anyone except his therapist. As a result, his behavior became increasingly cool toward the surviving son. When this son experienced the distancing from his father, he tried desperately to win back his father's affection. However, the more he tried, the more his behavior alienated his father. The therapist was finally able to help them both confront each other with very candid and painful feelings, and only after that confrontation did healing begin for both of them.

Lack of Support for Surviving Siblings

A final discriminating feature of sibling bereavement has to do with the support of surviving children by nonfamily members. In many cases bereaved parents receive more support from others than do their surviving children. People may focus their concern and love toward the parents, who have suffered this terrible loss of a child, and may overlook the feelings and concerns of the children. This is less likely to happen when a child experiences parental loss. With rare exceptions, the children in the Child Bereavement Study found that others outside the family were concerned about them and solicitous of their welfare. There is a tendency more readily to identify these children as bereaved than there is with children who lose a sibling to death.

SOME RESEARCH FINDINGS

I want to compare the findings of the Child Bereavement Study with those from several studies on sibling bereavement conducted by Betty Davies and Darlene McCown, who have done pioneering work on this subject (Davies, 1987, 1988a, 1988b, 1991; McCown, 1987; McCown & Pratt, 1985). Davies and McCown recorded the responses of 75 school-age children (50 families) to the death of a sibling during the first year of loss.

When comparing this study with the Child Bereavement Study (using the CBCL), we found that, overall, the loss of a sibling does not portend more emotional/behavioral problems than the loss of a parent. Furthermore, the percentage of children who could be termed "at risk" within the first year of bereavement is the same (approximately 25%), regardless of the type of loss. This means that in both groups, approximately three-quarters of the children were doing well or "making do" and did not need clinical intervention during the first year of bereavement.

However, a closer examination of the two groups, focusing on the age and gender of the children, did reveal some significant differences. In general, boys were more impacted by the loss of a parent than by the loss of a sibling. Preteen boys who lost a parent were more withdrawn, more anxious and depressed, and tended to show somatic symptoms more often than those who had lost a sibling. Both preteen and adolescent boys who lost a parent were also more likely to be placed in at-risk groups than their counterparts who lost a sibling.

In contrast, girls were more affected by the loss of a sibling. In particular, adolescent girls who lost a sibling showed disturbed behavior that included higher levels of anxiety and depression and more attention problems than adolescent girls who lost a parent. The differences between those who lost a sibling and those who lost a parent were especially high when comparing girls who had lost a sibling with those who had lost a father. It follows that girls who had lost a sibling, both preteen and adolescent, were more likely to be at risk than those who had lost a parent.

The reasons for these differences are not all that clear. The gender of the dead parent or of the dead sibling may offer some further clues as to the differences. Of the parentally bereaved boys, 75% had lost a father, while 25% had lost a mother. In the Boston study father loss was an important contributor to risk during the first year of bereavement. For the girls in the sibling study, the majority had lost a sibling of the same gender. It is clear, however, that the functioning of the bereaved family will contribute to the children's likelihood of being at risk. The functioning of the surviving parent plays a crucial role in the adaptation of parentally bereaved children to the loss (see Chapter 3). In like manner, family functioning will influence the adaptation of the child to the death of a sibling.

Do children who fall into the at-risk group come from the same families? Of the parentally bereaved, 21 out of 70 (30%) families had one or more children at risk during the first year of bereavement. Of these 21 families, 12 had *all* their children in the risk group. In the sibling bereaved group a smaller percentage of families (23%, consisting of 12 families) had at least one child in this risk group. However, 11 of these 12 families had *all* of their children at risk at some time during the first year after the death. Although a smaller percentage of families who lost a child have children at risk, when they do, this risk is more likely to affect a greater number of children in that family.

POINTS TO REMEMBER:
SIBLING VERSUS PARENTAL LOSS

- Overall, the loss of a sibling does not portend more emotional/behavioral problems than the loss of a parent during the first year of bereavement.
- Approximately one-quarter of the children fall into the at-risk group, regardless of the type of loss, during the first 6 months.
- In general, girls are more impacted by the death of a sibling and boys are more impacted by the death of a parent.
- Family influences that place children at risk are strong for both parentally and sibling bereaved children.
- Although a smaller percentage of families who lost a child have children at risk, when they do, this risk is more likely to affect a greater number of children in that family.

The Loss of a Parent by Divorce

How is the loss of a parent through divorce different from the loss of a parent through death? There are, to be sure, many similarities in the reactions of children to the breakup of the home via these two avenues, and similar adjustments that the family must make to accommodate to changes in family structure and role allocations. However, there are, again, some unique features that distinguish these two types of loss.

DISTINGUISHING FEATURES OF LOSS BY DIVORCE

Fantasies of Reunion

When a family breaks up through divorce, it is often difficult for the children to believe in the permanence of the situation. Fantasies of reunion are very common and are likely to continue for some time. Many children of divorce believe that, if they are just "good enough," the parent will return and the family will be reunited. When the various strategies that a child uses to bring about this reunion fail, a lower sense of self-esteem can result. Fantasies of reunion are less likely to be found among children who have lost a parent to death. The permanence and irreversibility of the loss are very real to most children, especially to children whose understanding of death is developed to the point that they grasp the abstractions of finality and irreversibility. Although a bereaved child may wish for the situation to be reversed, the belief in that option is short-lived and, in some respects, the knowledge of the permanence of loss helps the child and the family to get on with the task of rebuilding the family unit.

Difficulties in Mourning

Children whose parents are divorcing may feel the need to hide their mourning more than children who have a parent die. Mourning may not be supported by other family members or by the custodial parent, due to ongoing conflicts between parents. Also, mourning may not be acknowledged by these children of divorce because they have not made the loss real. Hopes for reuniting the family may keep the reality of the loss at a distance for some time. When a parent dies, the loss becomes real for the child very quickly. Even though the child struggles to maintain an ongoing relationship with the dead parent, the child realizes that the parent exists in another realm and will not return to make the family complete as it was before the death. The bereaved child is usually encouraged to grieve and is also more likely to find others with whom to share this grief.

Preloss Conflict

Divorce frequently occurs after a period of marital conflict and a deteriorating relationship between the parents. Such conflict between parents affects the ways in which children adjust to the divorce. A divorce occurring after several separations and reconciliations can feed reunion fantasies in these children, even years after the divorce. Although there can be marital conflict before a death, it usually is not the case. Many deaths occur suddenly, but when death is anticipated, the well parent is often drawn closer to the dying parent rather than the opposite. In fact, in our study one couple who was separated at the time of illness actually reunited after the illness developed and supported one another through the final months and weeks of life. However, it should be pointed out that some couples sustain a highly ambivalent relationship. When one member of such a couple dies, the surviving member may have a difficult bereavement, with anger and guilt being the predominant features of the grieving.

Loyalty Conflicts

In many divorce situations the ongoing tension between parents may continue for some time. The anger that spouses feel toward each other will be obvious to the children, particularly if each parent tries to paint a bleak picture of the other. Children in this situation often feel conflicted as each parent vies for the child's loyalty. Even when children are encouraged not to take sides, they often feel they must (Wallerstein & Blakeslee, 1989). Some children in this situation do not experience this pull and place their loyalty with one parent, often the custodial parent. However, many children in a divorce situation feel love and loyalty toward both parents and do not want to be caught in between parents in such a struggle. This conflict over loyalty adds to the stress felt by children of divorce. Also, if they side with one parent over the other, the children feel less hope that a reuniting of parents will ever occur. In bereaved families these struggles for loyalty are not present, making this a significant difference between these two types of loss.

The Ongoing Relationship with Children

The quality of the parent–child relationship has a powerful impact on childhood adjustment following both death and divorce. Parents in general, however, may be predisposed to behave in different ways to their children following death or divorce. For example, a bereaved parent, although stressed by the loss, may draw closer to the children and try to make up for the death of the other parent. In divorce, custodial parents may be more likely to see children as adding to their stress and may comment that the kids drive them crazy. However, these are not hard and fast differences; for example, tensions often run high between surviving parents and bereaved adolescents. In the Child Bereavement Study we have seen that children who have a poor relationship with the surviving parent are more likely to externalize their conflicts through acting-out behavior.

Choice and Anger

Divorce, more than death, is a matter of choice. The fact that one's parent has chosen to leave the family can leave the child feeling abandoned and less good about him- or herself and can lead to feelings of anger toward the person who left. Similar feelings of anger and rejection can also be found in the divorced parent who was left by his or her spouse, and the intensity of anger on the part of the custodial parent affects the adjustment of the child. When death occurs it is usually not the choice of the person who died and feelings of abandonment leading to anger are usually short lived. An exception to this would be parental suicide, where the choice to die often leads to high levels of guilt and anger on the part of the survivor, which may last for a long time (Worden, 1991).

Responsibility for the Breakup

It is common for children to assume personal responsibility for the breakup when divorce occurs. In trying to understand why the divorce happened, children often believe that they are part of the cause (Healy et al., 1993). Feelings of self-blame are stronger when children are caught in the struggle between their two parents. Children may feel that if they had just done something more, such as being better behaved, or not done something, the divorce would not have occurred. This sense of personal responsibility can lead to feelings of guilt and culpability. Although it is possible to find guilt and self-blame in children whose parent has died, this phenomenon is less common in a death situation. In the Boston study we only found 12% of the children who were grappling with some sense of responsibility over the death during our 2 years of follow-up.

Community Support

In general, community support is more available to bereaved families than to divorcing families. It is easier to feel compassion for children who have lost a parent to death than to divorce. Frequently, bad behavior in bereaved children is excused by others, for after all, the child's mother or father has died. When a child from a divorced family shows bad behavior, people may respond more negatively by saying, "No wonder she is a troublemaker, she comes from that broken family." In school the death of a parent is frequently acknowledged in the classroom by the teacher. The same is rarely the case when the family is undergoing divorce.

Wallerstein and Blakeslee (1989) found fewer than 10% of the children in their study had any adult speak to them sympathetically as the divorce unfolded.

Financial Struggles

After a divorce, money is often used as a weapon between the spouses. There are numerous examples of fathers who fail to pay alimony or child support, thus leaving the family in destitute circumstances. In some divorced families repeated court appearances over child support are the norm. Conflicts over money are a way to express anger at one's former spouse. This creates financial strains for the family and provides an avenue for ongoing conflict between parents, which takes its toll on the children. When a parent, especially a father, dies, the bereaved family may experience some financial decline. This decline can affect both the family and the surviving children, with the impact being greatest on adolescent children. However, money is rarely used as a weapon in bereaved families. Also, other monies often become available through pensions, insurance policies, and supplemental income sources. In fact, the government will step in and provide money to bereaved families with minor children through provisions of the Social Security Act. Such financial resources are not available to the divorced family. There is one negative scenario that may arise in more dysfunctional bereaved families receiving Social Security income. Adolescents in these families may feel that such insurance, because it is designated for the children, is theirs to spend as they like, and this can cause family friction.

Feeling Different

More children will experience the loss of a parent through divorce than through death. It is estimated that 20% of children will experience family divorce before age 18, whereas only an estimated 5% of children will experience parental death before that age. The main implication of this difference has to do with social relationships. Children, especially adolescents, do not want to be or appear different than their peers. Bereaved children, being fewer in number, run a higher risk of feeling odd or strange than do divorced children. In the Boston study 25% of the children were given a difficult time by other children at some point during the 2 years for not having both parents, and one-third of the children reported they felt strange among their peers for not having both parents. Some bereaved children acknowledged that they would have chosen for their parents to divorce, rather than for one parent to die. For example, one elementary school boy whose father was murdered said of boys from divorced families, "At least the other kids have fathers, whether they are living with them or not."

Fears for the Future

A major concern for children of divorce is whether or not this will be their own fate in future relationships. Data show that children from divorced families are more likely to end up divorced than children from intact families. Children of divorce fear repeating their parent's mistakes (Wallerstein & Blakeslee, 1989). Bereaved children are less likely to have such a concern. On the other hand, the death of one's parent makes death real for the child and may increase the child's personal death awareness (Worden, 1976). Concerns for their own mortality and possible fears accompanying this concern will be more prominent for bereaved children than for children of divorce.

Parental Dating Behavior

Although there are exceptions, divorced parents usually begin dating earlier than bereaved parents. In the Boston study only 12% of bereaved parents dated early, and these tended to be more depressed than parents who dated later (Worden & Silverman, 1993). Regardless of when dating begins, it can pose problems for some children. Dating in bereaved families, although not always comfortable, tends to be more acceptable for the children than in divorced families. One reason for this difference is the reunion fantasies often found among children of divorce. If the parent is dating or moving toward remarriage, this dashes any hope for the possible reuniting of the family. On the other hand, although bereaved children may experience some discomfort when a parent dates due to issues of loyalty to the dead parent, many are supportive of their surviving parent. One 4-year-old, eager to replace his dead father, asked his mother if they could go to the "daddy store" to get a new daddy. She informed him with a smile that it was not that easy. Bereaved parents who had a good marriage tend to be more reluctant about dating, for fear that they will not meet someone of equal quality to share their life with. Such was the case for the mother of this 4-year-old boy.

Family Restructuring

When a family experiences either death or divorce, some restructuring of the family is necessary in order for it to continue to function effectively (Bowen, 1978; Hetherington, 1993). There are several features in a divorce situation that tend to make this more difficult when compared to a death situation. One feature, mentioned earlier, is the persisting fantasy that reunion is possible. If it is possible to go back to what was, one will resist moving forward toward a restructured family. A second feature has to do with the continued involvement of both parents with the family. When the relationship is acrimonious and tensions high, these dynamics interfere with any restructuring. Challenges for restructuring may be found in the bereaved family but, on the whole, this task seems to be easier for bereaved families than divorced families. The reality of this need to regroup is clearer to all concerned and, although there may be a strong emotional tug to have the dead person back, the realization that this won't happen eventually hits everyone and the family moves forward with restructuring and new role allocations.

Children's Intimate Relationships

A final unique feature comes to us from the research of Mavis Hetherington (1972) and has to do with the way that girls who have experienced father absence relate to men in their lives. Using various research settings, Hetherington and colleagues have found that girls who have lost a father through divorce are much more flirtatious with a male stranger introduced into the research environment than are girls whose fathers died. The latter are more quiet and withdrawn around male strangers than are girls from divorced families. These daughters of widows showed more inhibition, rigidity, avoidance, and restraint around these males than daughters of divorcees. Hepworth and colleagues (1984) found that a group of college students with parental death, as a group, were more hesitant about intimate relationships. Persons with parental divorce generally showed accelerated courtship patterns.

SOME RESEARCH FINDINGS

The best comparisons between the effects of parental loss through divorce versus death can be made if large groups of children with these two losses are followed over time and assessed using the same measures. However, there are few, if any, studies of this type. Therefore, I want to review some of the recent literature on children of divorce and compare certain findings with findings from the Child Bereavement Study. It should be noted, however, that findings on children of divorce are not always consistent and these inconsistencies are due to some of the same methodological limitations as those outlined for the bereavement literature in the introduction to this book.

Blame for Parental Loss

As mentioned earlier, blame for the loss of a parent is one of the key features of loss through divorce. Healy and colleagues (1993) studied over 100 preadolescent children from divorced families and looked at the frequency of self-blame feelings about the parental separation. At 6 months after the separation about one-third of the children expressed such feelings. By 1 year later the figure had dropped to 20%. These feelings of self-blame were strongest in children who felt caught in a struggle between the two divorcing parents. Children with these feelings of guilt had lower self-esteem on the Harter (1979) inventory and more behavioral problems on the CBCL.

Self-blame was less frequent in our group of bereaved children than in the children of divorce group. Looking at the preadolescent group for comparability and using similar time frames, the self-blame figures for the bereaved group were 5% at 4 months and 7% at 1 year. Similar percentages were found in the adolescent group.

In the total bereaved sample feelings of guilt were not associated with lower self-esteem at either time point. They were associated with more emotional/behavioral problems at the 1-year time point but not at 4 months. Because death is quite a different phenomenon than divorce, it is not surprising to find more self-blame in the divorced group than in the bereaved group.

Gender Differences

Several studies of divorced families have found that boys had more difficulties after a divorce than girls (Doherty & Needle, 1991; Kelly, 1993; Shaw et al., 1993). Key correlates of this difficulty are the marital conflict between parents and the problems of parenting. In one study girls showed more negative reactions prior to the separation but not after the divorce. For boys the opposite occurred; they demonstrated more ill effects after the divorce but not prior to the separation. These gender differences tend to appear early following the divorce and are not as striking when one follows divorced children over time (Kelly, 1993; Wallerstein, 1991).

In the group of bereaved children there were some gender differences but fewer than might be expected. Neither boys nor girls showed more emotional/behavioral problems on the CBCL, nor were there significant gender differences relating to self-esteem and self-efficacy. Gender differences were, however, found on anxiety measures and school performance. In the early months after the death, girls were more concerned about their own safety and that of their surviving parent than were boys. Boys, on the other hand experienced more learning difficulties than did girls. All in all, poor adjustment to bereavement was found among both genders and depended to a great extent on the functioning of the surviving parent and on the stability of the home environment.

Academic Difficulties

More academic deficits have been found in children of divorce than among control children. Mulholland and colleagues (1991) found that children whose parents had divorced showed significant performance deficits in academic achievement, as reflected by grade point average and scholastic motivation, when compared to children from intact families. Such differences were not attributed to differences in social class or intellectual ability. Brisnaire et al. (1990) found a similar marked decrease in academic performance following parental separation, something that continued to be evident 3 years following the divorce. Looking at younger children whose parents had divorced, Hoyt and associates (1990) found more school adjustment problems in the divorced group than in demographically matched children.

Learning problems were experienced by a fifth of the bereaved children shortly after the death, and these were more likely to be experienced by boys than girls. However, one of the most significant findings from the Boston study was the lack of difference in learning problems when comparing the bereaved children with their matched controls 1 and 2 years following the death of the parent. Although learning difficulties continued for approximately 15% of the bereaved children into the first and second years of bereavement, this figure does not exceed the percentage of learning difficulties found in the nonbereaved matched control children. It appears that ongoing learning problems may be greater for the divorced group than the bereaved group and, if this is true, it is probably due to ongoing conflicts in the divorcing family. The Child Bereavement Study showed that children who experience many daily life changes and who feel less in control over what happens to them are more likely to experience learning difficulties and problems with concentration than are children with a more stable homelife and a greater sense of personal empowerment (see Chapter 4).

Early Adolescence

Hetherington (1993), presenting findings from the Virginia Longitudinal Study of Divorce and Remarriage, found that children who were in early adolescence when their parents divorced had a particularly difficult time in adapting to these family changes. This same group also had the most difficulty in adapting to parental remarriage. Reasons for this have to do with the developmental tasks associated with this stage of life.

We looked at the data from the Boston study to see if children whose parent died when they were early adolescents had significantly different adjustment and behavioral patterns than children who were younger or older when a parent died. We found that they did not appear to have significantly different scores on a number of outcome measures used in the study. This was true regardless of the assessment time point. However, children who were in early adolescence at the time of their parent's death did show more aggression during the second year than children who were older or younger at the time of death. This difference in aggressive behavior was not significant at earlier assessments but began to appear during the second year. This may be an artifact or it could be one of the late effects of bereavement. The latter possibility is supported by the fact that aggression in the bereaved adolescents was greater than that of their matched counterparts at that point in time.

Conflict with Parents

Interparental conflict has been identified as an important correlate of adjustment to divorce (Portes et al., 1992; Forehand et al., 1991). Portes and colleagues found that parental conflict and animosity led to higher levels of withdrawal, anxiety, and depression in children of divorce. Forehand and colleagues found that high levels of interparental conflict in divorced families were associated with parent–adolescent conflicts and high levels of such conflict led to poorer adjustment in these adolescents.

We looked at the bereaved children and found a similar correlation. When the entire group of adolescents was examined 2 years after the death, there was a strong association between having a poor relationship with the surviving parent and external-izing conflicts through acting-out behavior. This finding is similar to that of Forehand and colleagues (1991), who found that the parent–adolescent relationship was the best predictor of adolescent functioning in children of divorce.

POINTS TO REMEMBER:
LOSS BY DIVORCE VERSUS DEATH

• More school-age children will lose a parent to divorce than lose a parent to death.

• There are important differences in the experience of bereaved children and divorced children that will influence outcomes.

• Boys have more difficulty after a divorce and less after parental death.

• Self-blame for the loss is higher in divorced children than it is in bereaved children.

• Learning difficulties may be higher for divorced children than for bereaved children.

• Parental loss for children in early adolescence will pose problems for both loss groups.

• Parent–child conflict significantly affects adjustment in both loss groups.

HOW WE CAN HELP
BEREAVED CHILDREN

Counseling
and Intervention Issues

Our research has shown that not all bereaved children need or would necessarily profit from grief counseling. In fact, many bereaved children do well without any special intervention at all. Yet, children who lose a parent to death obviously suffer and have much to cope with. Their grief elicits a caring response from teachers, mental health providers, and others who want to help. In this chapter I want to look at ways in which responsible adults can meet the needs of bereaved children. Addressing certain basic needs, along with early screening, can help to minimize the possibility of children developing more serious problems. However, adults should also be aware that those children who do show extreme responses to the death of their parent need professional evaluation. Therefore, I want also to address in this chapter certain "red-flag" behaviors that may indicate the need for professional referral.

People who write about intervention with bereaved children often fail to make an important distinction between interventions for bereaved children who have serious adjustment disorders and interventions for children who are merely struggling with adaptation to the loss. The diagnosis and treatment of children experiencing serious emotional/behavioral difficulties following a loss will be very different from the intervention offered to more adequately coping children to facilitate them through the expected tasks of mourning. This distinction is often blurred and it needs to be made clearer.

The training level of those doing intervention with bereaved children must also be an important consideration. Many support groups for bereaved children are sponsored by schools, churches, or hospices and may be led by people with little or no training in child therapy. This need not be a problem as long as these leaders are trained to recognize specific behavioral signs ("red flags") that indicate when a child should be referred for professional evaluation and possibly for treatment.

BEREAVEMENT NEEDS OF GRIEVING CHILDREN

Findings from the Child Bereavement Study illustrate that the course of children's adaptation to the death of a parent varies. Some children appear to be doing well at the time of the 2-year follow-up, whereas other children are having a more difficult adjustment. For some, difficulties arise around the time of the death, while for others, late adjustment problems begin to appear in the second year after the loss. Although styles of grieving vary, the needs discussed here pertain to most bereaved children, and meeting these needs becomes the focus for the intervention models and activities discussed in Chapter 10. Mental health professionals can help interpret these needs to parents of bereaved children and can develop specific interventions to address these needs. Bereaved children need the following:

Adequate Information

Children need information that is clear and comprehensible. We have already seen that a child's understanding of death depends on his or her ability to deal conceptually with abstractions, such as finality and irreversibility. This understanding also depends on previous experiences with deaths of other persons and animals. When children do not have sufficient information, they will make up a story to fill in the gaps. One girl knew only that her favorite uncle died, but was not told that the uncle died of AIDS. She made up an elaborate story about how he had eaten poisoned meat,

meat that had been nibbled on by a rat who had eaten some poisoned cheese, and that is why he died. Later, when she was told the facts, she was able to handle them and gave up her fantasy.

If at all possible, children should be informed about an impending death. They know something is taking place, even if they are not told directly. A lack of information can make a child feel anxious and less important; and in a worst-case scenario, the child can feel responsible for what is happening to the dying person. It is also helpful for children to have clear information about the cause of death because, without this, they can develop unrealistic fears about death and disease. They may wonder, "Will it happen to me?" Of special import is the issue of contagion. Helping them know that "Daddy died of cancer" and that they cannot "catch" cancer can be reassuring for some, particularly younger children.

Fears and Anxieties Addressed

Children need to know they will be cared for. The death of a parent often elicits a primitive anxiety that one will not survive without one's parent—this same fear can also be experienced by adults (Bowlby, 1980). Many children who lose one parent fear that the other will die too. In the Boston study there was a significant increase in this type of fear during the first year of bereavement. Not only do children fear for the safety of their one remaining parent, but they fear for their own safety as well. These fears need to be directly addressed by those attending to the needs of these children and the appropriate reassurances given.

Strength (1991) studied a group of bereaved children who experienced father loss and found that children who were given consistent discipline after parental death were less anxious than those for whom discipline became lax. There is a tendency to ease up on discipline after a parental death because the children are going through so much, and the surviving parent doesn't need one more thing to tax his or her limited energy. However, consistency in the application of appropriate discipline after a death can go a long way to reassure the child and to reduce anxiety. Limit setting is what children inwardly desire, and enforcing limits can make a child feel cared for and ultimately more secure.

Reassurance They Are Not to Blame

Bereaved children may wonder, "Did I cause it to happen?" These children need to know that they did not cause the death out of their anger or shortcomings. Children learn early that strong feelings can hurt another person, and sometimes they misconstrue these strong feelings as having contributed to their parent's death. For example, they may be angry at the person and then the person dies. Could the feelings have contributed to the death? This question may very well be on the minds of some children. Adolescents, in particular, can have ambivalent or coexistent love–hate feelings toward a parent. The child needs to know that negative feelings toward the deceased did not contribute to or cause the death.

There is a period in the development of children, when they are on their way to mastering their environment, known as the "magic years" (Fraiberg, 1959). During this time, usually around ages 4 and 5, children believe that they have superpowers to make things happen. If a loss occurs during this developmental stage, the child will be more likely to feel some sense of responsibility for the death. Giving children an opportunity to talk about their feelings for the deceased, both positive and negative, can help parents and counselors identify any problems of culpability that may need to be reality tested with the child.

Careful Listening

Children have fears, fantasies, and questions and need a person who will hear them out and not minimize their concerns. Emerson said, "A friend is someone before whom you can think aloud." Adults need such friends and so do children. Many of the questions that arise around a death are complex, and it is important not to give children superficial answers, even though this can be awkward for adults. Questions such as, "Can Grandma still pee?" or "Why does God need a dead cat in heaven?" can make adults feel uncomfortable, yet these should be heard and answered as valid queries.

The listener may be someone other than a parent. This can be especially true in the case of teenagers who are dealing with issues of separation from family as part of their own development.

These other listeners can be teachers, counselors, relatives, family friends, or parents of peers.

Validation of Individuals' Feelings

Feelings must be acknowledged and respected as valid. It is very easy to tell a child how he or she should feel, and the temptation increases as adults try to protect themselves against feeling helpless. At 2 years after the death, one-quarter of the children in the Boston study reported getting admonitions from family members to show more feeling, whereas another quarter said they were told to finish their grieving. This latter group included children who reported high levels of crying into the second year of bereavement.

Children need to express their thoughts and feelings in their own way. It is easy for a bereaved parent to forget this and to expect that each child will express grief in the same way or on a similar timetable. These parents need to be reminded that each child has a distinct personality and each had a different relationship with the deceased. What the deceased parent was to one child can be different from what he or she was to another. These differences in relationships depend primarily on the age and gender of the child and the parent's hopes and expectations for that child. Such differences in personality and in relationship will make for varying expressions of grief. Some children are more open with their thoughts and feelings, while others disclose less. This does not necessarily mean that they do not care for the deceased or that they are heading for some kind of emotional difficulty related to the death.

Help with Overwhelming Feelings

Children need help in dealing with emotions that are too intense to be expressed. The death of a parent can elicit very strong feelings, feelings that are too scary for the child to express directly or feelings that become displaced as aberrant behavior patterns. As shown by the Boston study, the most common feelings expressed by bereaved children are sadness, anger, anxiety, and guilt. Although there is a tendency for adults to want to protect bereaved children from such feelings associated with loss, especially when these feelings increase from moderate to intense levels, one cannot protect children from these feelings. However, one can help them express them in safer ways.

Play activities can be useful in providing such safety. Children can draw or sculpt in clay and through these media express the intensity of a feeling, such as anger, that may be difficult for them to verbalize. Writing activities can also help children who need to express regrets and guilt feelings that may linger after a death (see Chapter 10).

Involvement and Inclusion

Children need to feel important and involved before the death as well as afterward. The youngest children in the family are frequently those who feel the least important and involved. One way to address this is to include children in funeral planning and in the funeral itself. Parents often ask whether children should attend funerals. I believe that children over age 5 should be given the opportunity to decide whether or not they want to attend, but it should be an informed decision. If a child has not previously been to a funeral, he or she needs to be given explicit information about what will be seen and experienced—for example, adults crying, the body lying in an open casket, and any other information appropriate to the specific situation. Parents need to make this decision for younger children.

In my experience most children, when given the choice, will opt to attend; but preparation is required to make it an optimal experience. I have a friend who was not allowed to attend funerals when he was a small child. Finally he was old enough to attend but no one prepared him for the experience. He thought he was going to a social outing and was traumatized by what he saw. These memories remain even into his adult years. Children who do not want to attend should not be forced, nor should children be compelled to do something at the funeral they do not want to do, such as to touch or kiss the deceased.

Children can be asked if there is anything they would like to see buried with the person. Some of the children in our study drew pictures; wrote stories; or selected objects, photographs, or flowers that they wanted to be included in the casket with their dead parent. This experience seemed to be helpful for them and not traumatic.

Children, like adults, need rituals, but there are few rituals in our society that include children. Families can be encouraged to develop their own rituals around anniversaries of the loss, and around holidays, birthdays, or other times when it is appropriate to remember the deceased in a more formal way. Children are very creative and many who participated in our study wanted to, and did, have input about what was done on these occasions.

Continued Routine Activities

Children need to maintain age appropriate interests and activities. Children worry about whether they will have to attend school the day of the funeral, or who will accompany them to the bathroom. These and various other concerns are developmentally appropriate but they can be misunderstood by adults in the context of bereavement. It is axiomatic, but often overlooked, that a bereaved child is still a child and, as such, may do things that seem insensitive to adults. One mother returned from burying her husband and looked out into the yard to see her two children playing funeral with the two neighbor children. They had set up three chairs side by side—one child was on the chairs as the body, one was the preacher, and the two neighbor children were the mourners. She was very upset when she saw this, and she called to talk about her concerns. She needed to be reminded that children cope and communicate through play activity. The two neighbor children had not attended the service and her children were simply showing them what happens at a funeral.

Modeled Grief Behaviors

Learning theory tells us that modeled behavior is one of the most potent sources of learning. Children learn how to mourn by observing mourning behavior in adults. They need to be with adults who can model appropriate grieving. One way to ensure a good adaptation to a loss is for the adults to show children it is alright to remember the deceased and to discuss these memories, both good and bad, as well as to talk about what they will miss or not miss about the person. These shared reflections are one of the important benefits of a funeral. Encouraging children to think about, to remember, and to talk about the deceased is a rather simple but effective way that adults can influence the course of bereavement in children. When talking about the deceased, people naturally feel sad; sanctioning these sad feelings and sharing one's own sadness with the child is very important.

One does not necessarily need to develop elaborate interventions for teaching children how to cope with loss. The results of the Boston study show that children with high levels of self-efficacy usually have parents who use active and effective coping strategies. What is needed are adults who know what to do after a loss and who model this to the children. This not only teaches children important ways of coping, but encourages shared experiences that provide a supportive environment for the family to come together in the context of bereavement.

Opportunities to Remember

Children need to be able to remember and to memorialize the lost parent not only after the death but continuously as they go through the remaining stages of life. Silverman (1989) studied a group of college-age women who, at an earlier age, had lost a parent to death. These students reported that they were continually rethinking the loss and renegotiating their relationship to their dead parent as they matured from girls into women. What the parent was to the child at age 8 was different than what the parent would become when the child reached adolescence or adulthood.

There are various ways to help children memorialize their parent. Pictures and other objects belonging to the deceased can be useful reminders of who the person was and the things that were important in the relationship. Shared reminiscences in a family can also be helpful—some families seem to be more adept in doing this than others. If a bereaved parent remarries, it is important that the bereaved child be able to talk about and remember the dead parent, as well as to adjust to the relationship with the stepparent. Some children in the Boston study had a surviving parent who found it difficult to talk about their dead spouse. In such cases the children found they could have these shared reminiscences with their siblings or someone outside the family, even if their parent did not want to talk about the deceased.

IDENTIFYING CHILDREN
FOR PROFESSIONAL EVALUATION

The question of when to refer for professional evaluation has been addressed by Fox (1985), Grollman (1967), Webb (1993), Kliman (1968), and Osterweis et al. (1984), among others. Various behaviors have been identified that would indicate the need for professional evaluation by a child specialist. However, in the Child Bereavement Study we found that, while bereaved children show a variety of behaviors, many of the so-called "disturbed behaviors" are short lived and drop out on their own without any intervention. The focus should not be on the presence of a symptom or behavior but on its duration. If any of the following red-flag behaviors continue for several months, a professional evaluation should be warranted.

1. If the child has *persisting difficulty talking about the dead parent,* this can be a sign for further investigation. The emphasis here is on persisting difficulty. Some children are so uncomfortable when the conversation turns to the dead parent that they may leave the room. If this continues, check it out.

2. *Aggressive behavior* is not uncommon after a loss but should be monitored. If the aggressive behavior persists or takes the form of property destruction, then this child should be evaluated.

3. As with aggression, it is not uncommon for a child to feel *anxiety* after the death of a parent. A number of children in the Child Bereavement Study felt increasingly anxious about their surviving parent during the first year of bereavement. For most children this anxiety attenuates over time. However, if anxiety persists for the child, and especially if the child clings to the surviving parent or exhibits phobic behavior about going to school, then evaluation is warranted.

4. Some children express their grief through *somatic complaints* such as stomachaches, headaches, and the like. Most of these physical symptoms are self-limiting, but if a child experiences

prolonged bodily distress after a parent's death or if the child develops psychosomatic problems, then evaluation is in order. Occasionally a child will experience the exacerbation of a preexisting physical condition within the context of a loss and this, obviously, requires medical attention.

5. It is not uncommon for children to experience *sleeping difficulties* after the death of a parent. In the Child Bereavement Study 30% of the children experienced some kind of sleep disturbance during the first year of bereavement. Disturbances ranged from difficulty falling asleep to early morning awakening. If sleep disturbance persists for a number of months, the child should be evaluated by a professional. The same would hold true if the child experiences persisting nightmares.

6. *Eating disturbance* may be a sign of clinical depression, both overeating and not eating well. Eating behavior is so variable in children that this sign must be looked at with some caution—one must not rush to the conclusion that a problem exists. However, eating disturbances can arise in a bereavement context and persisting changes in eating patterns need to be watched and possibly evaluated.

7. One should be concerned when a child shows *marked social withdrawal* after a death, wanting to be by him- or herself, particularly when this pattern was not present prior to the death. This is not so worrisome in the short term, but if such behavior persists, it might be worthy of evaluation.

8. *School difficulties or serious academic reversal* can be a sign of poor adaptation to a loss. In the Boston study school difficulties were experienced by 20% of the children during the first year of bereavement but dropped to 15% during the second year. Persisting school difficulties should be seen as a red flag, possibly requiring further evaluation.

9. *Persistent self-blame or guilt* following a death should also lead to concern. Guilt, along with an overall sense of unworthiness, is often found in clinical depression and is sometimes the characteristic distinguishing depression from grief. Although grief and depression share many common features—such as dysphoria, low energy, and eating and sleeping problems—a pervasive sense of unworthiness is usually not present after a death and, if it is, usually points to clinical depression.

10. The child who is showing *self-destructive behavior* or who is expressing *a desire to die* should always be referred regardless of the length of time. Although this behavior is less common, it must be taken seriously. Some children miss their dead parent so much that they express a desire to die and to rejoin the lost parent. This may be more true of children with a less well-developed understanding of concepts related to death, such as finality and irreversibility. Children who have lost a parent to suicide may also think about this option for themselves. Some people are hesitant to ask children about their suicidal wishes, fearing that the question may plant the idea in the child's mind. However, this is not the case—a gentle inquiry is appropriate if one has any suspicions that such thoughts may be present. Simple questions like "Have you ever thought of hurting yourself?" or "Have you ever threatened or attempted to hurt yourself?" are often sufficient to open up a discussion of this important area.

It is difficult at times, even for clinicians, to assess when behavior is a normal response to loss and when it becomes pathological. One good example was presented by Wolfelt (1993) when he raised the question as to whether acting-out behaviors are related to normal grieving or to attention-deficit/hyperactivity disorder (ADHD). It's possible that some bereaved children who demonstrate acting-out behavior are inappropriately diagnosed as having ADHD and subsequently treated with Ritalin or other medication. Wolfelt suggests that clinicians who are evaluating acting-out behavior following a death consider that such behavior may be normal and may serve the child's survival needs. He suggests that this behavior may serve the following functions for such children:

- Expressing insecurity
- Expressing feelings of abandonment when losing a parent, leading to a self-fulfilling prophecy of being unloved
- Provoking punishment, as consistent discipline is a way to help children feel more secure
- Subtly alienating others in order to prevent future losses
- Countering their own personal death anxieties by proving, through hyperactivity, that they are still alive

- Externalizing internal feelings of grief, which build up and then explode

The clinician therefore needs to discriminate between the distractibility, impulsiveness, and hyperactivity that are part of the normal grieving process for some children and the criteria for ADHD listed in the fourth edition of the *Diagnostic and Statistical Manual of Mental Disorders* (DSM-IV; American Psychiatric Association, 1994). Clearly, even when acting-out or other behaviors are seen to be normal, these children have needs and conflicts precipitated by the loss that should be addressed by significant others.

Identifying red-flag behavior and referring for further evaluation is not the same process as the early screening and intervention described in the next section. In the identification of red flags, the behavior in question is currently present and provides the clue that the child should be targeted for further evaluation. The early screening approach, using the instrument found in Appendix B, identifies children that have high probability of emotional/behavioral difficulties 1 and 2 years after the death. Such difficulties may not be there at the time of early screening.

EARLY IDENTIFICATION
OF HIGH-RISK CHILDREN

There are essentially three ways to approach intervention with bereaved children. The first is to offer intervention to all of them. This approach assumes that losing a parent to death is a significant stressor for any child and that intervention can preclude negative effects from such a loss. However, our study of this community-based sample of bereaved school-aged children shows that only a third of the children fell into the risk category at any point during the first 2 years of bereavement. The other two-thirds appeared to be adjusting well to the death during this time period. Not only is this first approach not needed, it is not cost effective. Thus, with cost being a major concern in this time of shrinking healthcare dollars, this approach is not the best one.

A second approach to intervention with bereaved children is to wait until the child gets into difficulty and then offer intervention. This is a commonly used approach, but by definition requires that the child experience an observable level of emotional/behavioral distress before intervention is offered.

There is a third approach to intervention that comes out of the tradition of preventative mental health. This approach involves early screening to identify those most at risk and early intervention to preclude later negative sequelae from the loss. To develop a screening instrument one must follow over time a group of children who have not received intervention in order to identify those who make the poorest adaptation. Once these children are identified, variables gathered close to the time of death are used to discriminate those with poor adaptation from those with good adaptation. These predictor variables are then assessed in newly bereaved children, and intervention can be offered to those predicted to be at risk, with the expectation that early intervention will preclude poorer adaptation.

In the Child Bereavement Study we were able to identify those children with the poorest adaptation and to develop a screening instrument for early identification. The instrument consists of six items that describe key aspects of the child and surviving family, such as the number of children in the family under 12, the surviving parent's levels of stress and coping, the child's behavior, and other items. A more detailed description of the instrument, together with scoring information, can be found in Appendix B.

The needs of bereaved children listed above should be the basis of intervention with them. The next chapter outlines various models for intervention along with various activities to be used with bereaved children.

POINTS TO REMEMBER: COUNSELING AND INTERVENTION ISSUES

• Most bereaved children do not need special counseling. However, a third of the children have emotional/behavioral problems sufficient to warrant some type of counseling intervention during the first 2 years of bereavement.

• Those counseling bereaved children need to understand which behaviors are "red flags" and warrant further intervention.

• Bereaved children have 10 primary needs and intervention should address these needs.

• Acting-out behavior in bereaved children may be a part of normal grieving and not due to attention deficit or hyperactive disorders. Clinicians should be able to distinguish those behaviors that are normal from those portending a more serious disorder.

• Our preferred philosophy of intervention with bereaved children is to identify early those most in need through screening and to intervene. This approach is the most cost effective and falls into the tradition of preventative mental health.

Intervention Models
and Activities

The mental health professional interested in setting up an intervention program for bereaved children needs to select a model appropriate to the goals of that program and the setting in which it will take place. Each of the following models of intervention has its strengths and particular area(s) of focus. Many of the interventions deal with present relationships, both family and peer, focusing on the need for good communication and support. Others address particular tasks of mourning that have not yet been negotiated in adjustment to the loss, such as effective ways to remember and memorialize the deceased. Fundamental to each intervention model or program is the presence of a significant other who provides consistent support, reassurance, and information within a safe space in which people who have lost a family member to death can express their thoughts and feelings.

MODELS OF INTERVENTION
WITH BEREAVED CHILDREN

Peer Groups

Groups for bereaved children can be an effective model for intervention with several advantages. They can provide a safe supportive context in which children can express feelings without worrying about the presence of other family members. In a group children can receive support from both their peers and the leader. Contact with bereaved peers gives the child the reassurance that he or she is not alone in the experience of loss. Group intervention provides a place for the child to learn about death as well as a place to confront faulty beliefs about loss. In addition, group counseling can reach a larger number of children than either individual or family counseling and is, therefore, a cost-effective resource. Group interventions can also be readily adapted to school settings.

Peer support groups can be especially helpful for bereaved adolescents. As discussed, adolescent grief can be complicated by normal developmental struggles over dependence, autonomy, and issues of separating from parents. The Child Bereavement Study has shown that peer relationships are very important to the adolescent; most bereaved kids do not want to appear different or strange by crying or expressing sad affect in front of their friends. Consequently, adolescents may shut out avenues of support from both the surviving parent and friends. In a bereavement support group adolescents receive peer support from others who have sustained a similar loss. Gray (1989) found that students participating in bereavement support groups reported more support from peers at the completion of the group than they reported when the group began. Social support, in turn, affects emotional distress. Balk (1990), an expert on adolescent bereavement, found that bereaved adolescents who reported more social support had lower depression scores on the Beck Depression Inventory (1967) than those who reported less support.

Despite the advantages of social support, there are disadvantages to a group model. Groups are less well suited to deal with children who have severe or pathological reactions to the loss, and they do not address family issues directly. Although peer support is important, the home environment remains the most crucial influence on childhood bereavement. If the surviving parent is not adapting well to the loss, then the usefulness of peer support may be severely undercut.

Individual Counseling

A second intervention model uses individual counseling with bereaved children. Individual counseling frequently uses nondirective play activity in which children play with various toys and games and interact with the counselor. The assumption underlying this approach is that children process conflict and anxiety through play, imagination, and creative activity. The counselor uses these activities to explore the child's adjustment and to facilitate grieving within a safe context. Adjustment issues frequently explored include the child's ability to conceptualize death, the ability to form some type of lasting relationship with the deceased, and the child's present relationship to surviving family members.

In addition to nondirective play, counselors employing the individual counseling model may use guided imagery techniques to help children grieve (Bengesser, 1988; McIntyre, 1990). In a manner graduated for safety, children are asked to imagine specific scenes. The child can then interact with the person in the scenario. For example, the child may hold an imaginary conversation with the dead parent, saying what needs to be said, asking forgiveness, or expressing previously unsaid feelings. This is an effective way of completing unfinished business after the death. Scenes can also be modified and reworked with a different ending.

Art activities such as drawing are also appropriate to individual counseling and give children the opportunity to transform their loss creatively (McIntyre, 1990). Artistic expression may be easier for some children than verbal expression. Examples of art activities can be found on pages 162–163.

There are several advantages to an individual model of counseling and therapy. It is the treatment of choice for children experiencing complicated bereavement resulting in serious behavior and emotional disturbance, as these children may be less well suited for group intervention. Individual counseling offers the bereaved child an environment of emotional security and stability at a time when it may be difficult for the surviving parent to provide these conditions. A consistent emotional environment may help the child to sustain the process of mourning when it would otherwise be disrupted. This model also provides the child with a supportive adult relationship. A stable relationship between a child and any significant adult figure is related to greater resilience and better social adjustment in bereaved children (Altschul & Pollock, 1988; Garmezy, 1987; Zambelli & DeRosa, 1992).

There are three main limitations to the individual counseling model. First and foremost, it is the least cost effective in terms of resources, both of money and personnel. Second, it does not address directly the interactions between the bereaved child and the surviving parent. Finally, it does not focus on the overall functioning of the family system, an important component underlying some aberrant behavior resulting from the death of a parent.

Family Interventions

Family intervention is designed to give bereaved children an opportunity to work through their grief within the context of the family. It allows family members to talk together about the death and to readjust the family as a working system after the loss. Some family interventions focus primarily on *communication,* while others focus on the changes in roles and structure needed for *family readjustment.* Still others focus on *problem solving* and dealing with practical issues of family life affected by the death.

Communication

Open communication among family members is important. It enables the family to have a shared understanding of the death, provides social support within the family system itself, and allows the child to receive support from the surviving parent. In family intervention the counselor can model effective communication and resolution skills for the bereaved family. This often helps family members resolve unfinished business regarding the death on their own.

Warmbrod (1986) believes that communication between children and their surviving parent should be the emphasis in family intervention, because sharing grief between the child and parent within therapy increases the awareness that a family still exists. The surviving parent may also be taught to assist the bereaved child's grieving. Rosenthal (1980) believes that surviving parents who are unable to communicate grief can hinder the bereavement adaptation of their children. He assumes that if a surviving parent is unable to communicate about the loss, children will learn not to communicate about the loss as well. This cuts the child off from the family and forces the child to grieve outside the home. Improving family communication can release children from acting out these issues and can target denial within the family.

Black and Urbanowicz (1987) have attempted to study the effectiveness of communication-focused family intervention. They looked at 45 families in which 83 children suffered the loss of a parent. The authors designed a brief six-session family intervention to encourage the expression of grief and family communication about the dead parent. Families were assessed before the intervention and for a period of 2 years following the intervention. The authors report that intervention was effective in shortening the period of problems following bereavement, and they conclude that the treatment group benefited. However, their conclusions must be viewed with caution due to a high subject attrition rate at the 2-year follow-up (Black & Urbanowicz, 1987).

York and Weinstein (1980–1981) advocate a video technique for enhancing family communication. Bereaved families are shown a videotape of a family openly discussing the death of one of its members. They found that this increased the number of discussions of the death over that found in bereaved families who were not shown the video.

Family Readjustment

Family counselors who make family readjustment the goal of intervention will pay particular attention to the roles played by the deceased parent and his or her unique relationships with family members. The family must adjust to the loss of these roles and relationships and restore a homeostatic balance to the system (Bowlby-West, 1983). A number of shifting roles and new coping situations will occur in response to this structural change, some of which may be maladaptive. Usually a family's reshifting of roles represents an adequate adjustment to the loss. However, when the process of adjustment goes poorly, family dysfunction can crystallize and the bereaved child may show symptoms of this dysfunction (Gelcer, 1983). One example of this would be asking an older child to play the disciplinarian role previously played by the dead parent. The child may take on the role but may also feel anger over this new responsibility and display acting-out behavior (Krell & Rabkin, 1979). Poor family adjustment results when role assignments have little to do with the child's actual capabilities.

In an earlier work (Worden, 1991) I point out how a family

adjusts as a system to the loss of a parent. Families must restructure roles to fill the absence of the dead parent's roles and these roles must be assigned, negotiated, and accepted. Previous dyadic and triangular alliances (the emotional bonding patterns between two and three family members) must shift into a new equilibrium. Identifying these roles and alliances and encouraging healthy re-structuring is a task of family intervention (Bowen, 1978).

Some family counselors approach childhood bereavement apart from family systems theory but still use the family as their target unit. These approaches characteristically are brief and focus primarily on the bereavement experience. For example, Sills et al. (1988) use a Transactional Analysis approach with bereaved families in a six-session format. They spend two sessions assessing the family and its interaction patterns, two on facilitating grief, and two on grief resolution. The authors identify family self-images and con-front long-standing patterns of familial interaction in an effort to increase appropriate communication about the deceased.

Problem Solving

Family interventions can also address the coping or adjustment of the surviving parent. Poorly adjusted bereaved children come from families with poorly adjusted surviving parents. In an earlier study Van Eerdewegh and colleagues (1985) matched bereaved and nonbereaved school-age children and found that the mental health of the parent was a contributing factor to the mental health of the child. In the Child Bereavement Study children who adjusted poorly to the death tended to come from homes in which the surviving parent reported many life changes, was depressed, was less able to mobilize support from the community, and saw personal coping as inadequate. These children also reported many disrup-tions and arguments in their homes.

Family intervention can include more than one bereaved family in a session at a time. Greaves (1983) uses a multifamily grief counseling approach to improve communication. Multifa-mily groups include two or more bereaved families who meet together for mutual support, education, and sharing. These groups primarily confront family myths—those shared beliefs and practices within a family system that may inhibit appropriate grieving. If the family myth consists of the belief that it is not alright to talk about the deceased at home, this will leave members unable to support one another. Also, it is assumed that if a loss within the family is not adequately mourned, the effects of the loss can be felt for generations (Detmer & Lamberti, 1991; Paul & Grosser, 1965).

There are several advantages of family interventions. They provide a setting in which a child's grief can be processed naturally. Both the child and family can be assessed and treated, with gains introduced instantly into the home, enabling the family to operate as a natural support system and as a possible barrier to poor adjustment to the loss. Family intervention directly addresses some of the risk factors identified by Silverman and Worden (1992), Altschul and Pollock (1988), and Van Eerdewegh and colleagues (1982), particularly the adjustment of the surviving parent. In this context the parent's availability and supportiveness for the child can be assessed and facilitated. Replacement roles and pathological patterns created to restore family homeostasis can be directly assessed and confronted, and the child's role in the "new" family structure can be addressed. All members are obviously affected by the death of a family member and a readjustment must be made in which roles are healthfully reallocated and the expression of grief freely allowed. Also, there is some empirical evidence that family interventions may be effective (Black & Urbanowicz, 1987).

There are some disadvantages in using family interventions with bereaved children. Family interventions, like individual interventions, may be less cost effective than others such as group intervention. Practitioners may overlook or may not choose to focus on the child's intrapsychic reactions to the loss, if these reactions do not arise spontaneously in family treatment. Family therapies that do not assess the beliefs, meanings, and reactions of the individual child may miss important information, particularly when dealing with complicated bereavement. Finally, there is simply less focus on the individual bereaved child when emphasis is directed to the entire family. In this type of intervention for bereaved families, the counselor must let the child be heard and must address the child's needs. The surviving parent's needs are important but must not monopolize the intervention.

Combination Models

Combination models of intervention unite group, individual, and family models in various ways. The rationale for these combined models is to increase the effectiveness of intervention and to include more members of the family if specific family therapy is not done.

One combined intervention offers supportive counseling to the surviving parent in the belief that a parent who has accepted and adjusted to the loss of a spouse greatly reduces the risk of a poor grief reaction in the child. A better adjusted parent can provide a more supportive context for the child's grieving. Parent education about how to respond to the child and his or her experience with the death can also be helpful (Fox, 1985; Gardner, 1983). Joint sessions with the parent and child or with the entire family can follow this work.

Siegel et al. (1990) proposed such an intervention. Their program is educational and adopts a parent guidance model that indirectly targets children through interventions with the surviving parent. These parents are provided with the support, knowledge, and insight that will enable them to promote conditions that foster their children's grief work. Within this program, the surviving parents are trained to maintain the consistency in and stability of the child's environment, to allow a context for the free expression of grief, and to remain competent in dealing with the care and support of their children despite their own grief.

Muir et al. (1988) have also designed an intervention for the surviving parent. In response to studies showing that the surviving parent's unresolved mourning interferes with a child's capacity to mourn, these clinicians use an intervention program that integrates family and individual treatment. They assess the child, the surviving parent, and the home situation, and then provide treatment to both the child and the parent. The goal of this intervention is to preserve or restore family cohesiveness and ensure the surviving parent's psychological well-being, while at the same time attending to the child's individual distress. This intervention thus targets the child's family environment, the meaning of the loss and the distress of the death to the child, and the well-being of the surviving parent.

Berlinsky and Biller (1982) also endorse a combined individual child and family therapy approach. They state that this combination of family and individual treatment allows the child a corrective mourning experience (Paul & Grosser, 1965) and allows the family to stabilize its functions.

Zambelli et al. (1988) have used a combination of group counseling with bereaved children and simultaneous support groups for the children's parents. Their group counseling for children consists largely of art therapy, while the bereaved parent receives education and support from peers regarding the loss. The grief process is facilitated within a supportive social context for both the child and the parent. In like manner, Schwartz-Borden (1986) designed an intervention program in which both children and surviving parents are seen in simultaneous supportive groups designed to facilitate the expression of grief. Counselors lead the groups, paying close attention to age-related issues.

The well-known Dougy Center in Portland, Oregon, also combines intervention approaches. The Center runs groups for bereaved children that encourage the children to "play out" their grief in a nondirective fashion as well as to interact with peers during process times within the group. Surviving parents meet in their own groups at the same time as the children's groups in order to support one another. Such an approach appears to be successful (Smith, 1991).

ACTIVITIES FOR INTERVENTION

Whatever model is chosen for intervention, specific activities, selected as relevant to the age of the child, can be used to meet those needs of bereaved children outlined in the previous chapter. The activities listed below are intended to help bereaved children in several ways:

- They help facilitate the various tasks of mourning.
- They provide children with acceptable outlets for their feelings, including ways to address their fears and concerns.
- They help children get answers to their questions.
- They help counter misconceptions that children have about the death.

- They make discussions of death a normal part of the child's experience, something that may not be happening at home or in other settings.

Here are some specific activities listed by category.

Art Activities

Art activities are easy to use because children, from early ages on, love to draw and to express themselves with crayons, paper, and sculpting with clay. These expressive activities have several advantages. Children can remember their pain in measured amounts and attend to one aspect of the death at a time. Sadness and other feelings can be shared with an interested adult, and some of the inner turmoil a child may be experiencing can be put into words. Completing an art project can also provide the child with an important sense of mastery, something that death challenges in us all.

Drawing

When using drawing as a bereavement activity, the counselor provides the child with the materials and may suggest subjects. Here are some ideas:

- Draw something you worry about.
- Draw something that makes you mad.
- Draw yourself and write words that describe yourself.
- Draw your favorite memory of your dead father, mother, sister, and so forth.
- Draw a recent dream that you have had.
- Draw the ugliest picture you can.
- Draw your family.
- Draw yourself before your parent died; draw yourself now.
- Draw something that scares you.

To make these art activities effective, the children must be encouraged to share their pictures and to talk about them. In a group setting pictures can be shared with another child, then with a group of four children, and finally with the whole group.

Some counselors take a different approach when using art work with bereaved children. They will not suggest a specific topic for a drawing but will give materials to the children and then play various types of background music (harsh, peaceful, lively). Children are then free to draw whatever they like, but there is usually a relationship between the themes of the drawings and the flavor of the music being played. Again, these drawings, and the feelings elicited, can be shared with the counselor or the entire group.

Clay Modeling

The use of clay is another effective way to involve bereaved children in art activities. In both drawing and in clay sculpting, the colors selected by a child may reflect his or her feeling tone. For example, the use of red may reflect angry feelings or blue, sad feelings. However, I would caution lay counselors from making deep psychological interpretations of the children's work and would suggest that they ask the children themselves how and what they are feeling. When using clay, the counselor can either suggest things to be sculpted, such as "create your anger," or let children sculpt against the background of music or simply on their own.

Puppet Activities

Children of all ages like to use puppets, which appeal to adults as well. Manipulating a puppet removes children from speaking for themselves and gives them an opportunity to project onto the puppet thoughts and feelings that may be difficult for them to own. It offers a safe distance but is still a very energized activity. Puppets can be provided by the counselor or they can be made by the children. Small paper bags that fit easily over the child's hand can be drawn on, with holes for the eyes and mouth. Some counselors have the child make a puppet that looks like each of the family members, including the deceased parent. Letting each of these family members interact in the form of puppets can give the counselor, as well as the child, important insights into thoughts, feelings, and misperceptions that are current for the child.

Writing Activities

In addition to art activities, the various needs of the bereaved child can be facilitated through a number of writing activities.

Journaling

Writing journals is an activity that appeals to and can be used with older children. The child is provided with a notebook and is encouraged to write down feelings, thoughts, and questions about the lost loved one. The child can also be encouraged to write down dreams, especially dreams that involve the deceased. Some children enjoy writing poems and these can be written in their journals. Counselors should be aware of privacy issues associated with this activity and should obtain the permission of the child if this material is to be shared with others.

Letters

Writing letters to the deceased can also be used, but the counselor must use discretion here. One does not want to confuse the child whose concepts of death do not include finality and irreversibility, or the child who believes that the parent or sibling is just "away for a while" and will be returning. When appropriate, letters can include things the child wanted to say to the parent, such as statements of caring or asking forgiveness for something not done or said before the death. These letters can be kept, sent heavenward in a balloon, buried in the ground, or expedited in a number of different ways. Practitioners familiar with Gestalt psychotherapy often have clients write letters to deceased individuals in order to complete unfinished business. Letters written in the present tense and directed toward the lost loved one can be more effective in the completion of these issues than merely talking with the counselor about them.

Lists

Some children like to make lists, which can then be shared with the counselor or members of a group. Lists are especially useful in assessing the children's understanding about death and the specifics regarding their own loss. Lists can also be a useful tool in identifying and discussing misinformation. Children can list the facts about their parent's death, and they may list ideas such as that the dead can see or hear, that the body cannot move, and when you die you have a funeral. Then the children can make lists of their "fantasies" about the parent's death. They may list that "he or she can still see me, he or she will be mad if I do poorly in school," and so forth. Discussions can then take place regarding the reality underlying these facts and fantasies.

Memorials

Children can be asked to design a memorial service for their parent. This may include the activities, location, and things they want said about their parent that will help them and others remember. This is often an activity that captures the imagination of children, although younger children may not be able to do this without assistance. As mentioned earlier, we asked the children in the Child Bereavement Study to redesign their deceased parent's funeral 2 years after the death. More than half of the children gave us a redesigned service. A similar activity asks the child what he or she would write on the parent's memorial marker, a phrase that would epitomize the life of the parent, or something that would communicate to others who the parent was.

Memory Book

Those who have attended my workshops on bereaved children know that I am enthusiastic about the use of the memory book. It combines the best of both writing and art activities. Essentially, a memory book is a scrapbook of memories about the deceased. In it children can place pictures they have drawn, stories they have written, and photographs they have selected. The memory book may contain artifacts from activities that the child remembers doing with their dead parent, and things that they will want to remember in the future. One child wanted to focus on his trip to Disney World, so he wrote a story about the trip, drew some pictures, and cut and pasted some of the photographs that the family had taken on the trip. Other children in this same family had other remembrances that were special for them and included materials in the book that reflected these particular memories.

I believe that the memory book is best done as a family activity, with each child and other family members contributing to the book. It can provide a way for families to ensure memories and to talk about the deceased with each other. Another important advantage of the memory book is that it gives children something to revisit and review as they move through the various developmental stages of their life. Many bereaved children have the fear that they will forget their lost parent. A memory book can give them something concrete to hold onto and to ensure that this won't happen. Younger children who had a more limited contact with their deceased parent can learn more about the dead parent as they grow and their interest in who their parent was changes.

Storytelling Activities

There are a number of good books that deal with grief and bereavement written for children of various age levels. Two of my favorites are *The Fall of Freddie the Leaf,* written by Leo Buscaglia, and *Aarvy Aardvark,* written by Donna O'Toole. These stories can be read to bereaved children and then discussed individually or in a group. Children can tell how the story made them feel. Another good way to open up a dialogue is to have them draw their personal reactions to the story. A more indirect approach to feelings is to read the story to the children and then ask them how the bereaved character in the story might have been feeling.

Counselors can also ask children to write a story about their own loss and then share this story with the counselor or with the group. This combines the activities of storytelling and writing. A list of books for bereaved children, divided by appropriate age categories, can be found in Wass and Corr (1982).

Games

Games are very useful in group settings. Children love games of all kinds and, because it is "only a game," it becomes easier for bereaved children to express taboo feelings and beliefs. Games in which all the children participate are a good way to normalize discussions of death. Games can also give children new ways of coping and relating to other children. There are many different kinds of games suitable for use with bereaved children. I have listed several below to give you a sense of the variety of possibilities.

Five Faces (Jewett, 1982)

Children are given crayons and five blank cards. They are asked to draw five different faces representing five different feelings—sad, glad, mad, scared, and lonely. Children love competition, so the leader can ask who can draw the saddest face. After each child has completed his or her five faces, the cards are shuffled into a face-down pile. Each child gets an opportunity to select a card and then tells the group about an experience that made them feel like the feeling portrayed on the card. As an alternative procedure, completed cards can be shuffled and five cards dealt to each child. When a child gets two cards representing the same feeling, he or she tells the group about experiences associated with that feeling.

Question Box (Segal, 1984)

Each child in the group is handed slips of paper on which they can write their questions about death or funerals. There should be one question per slip. Question slips are then collected and placed in a box. Each child is given the opportunity to select a question, to read it to the group, and to lead a discussion on the question.

It's Not Fair When . . . (Jewett, 1984)

Each child is given a small box, such as a shoe box. Going around the circle, each child is given an opportunity to complete the sentence "It's not fair when . . . ," while slamming the box down onto the floor. After each child has participated, the boxes are stacked in a pile and knocked down by the children. The goal of this activity is to help the children to connect their actions with their words, and to find an acceptable way to express their anger.

Changes

Each child is given a piece of paper and crayons and is asked to divide the page by a vertical line. On the left side the child is asked to draw his or her family before the death. On the other side the child is asked to draw the family since the death. These pictures are shared with the rest of the children in the group.

The Weather Inside

Children are given paper and crayons and asked to draw what the weather was like on the day of their parent's funeral. After they do this, they are asked to draw what the weather was like inside of them on that day. These drawings are then discussed.

Show and Tell

This is not really a game but is similar to the "show and tell" activity often used in school settings. Children are encouraged to bring to the group a picture of their dead parent or some object that is associated with a special memory of their parent. Each child, in turn, is given the opportunity to share these objects and pictures.

Feeling Circle

Each child is given a page with a large circle drawn on it. Children are asked how they are feeling today and then are asked to select a colored crayon that represents that feeling. The children color the circle and write the name of the feeling or feelings under it. As an alternative, circles can be drawn on a page and children with multiple feelings they want to express can color different circles to represent their various feelings.

I encourage those who counsel bereaved children to make up their own activities. If one understands the tasks of mourning and the bereavement needs of grieving children, then one can make up activities that will help facilitate these tasks and meet the children's needs.[1]

POINTS TO REMEMBER:
INTERVENTION MODELS AND ACTIVITIES

- There are four intervention models commonly used with bereaved children and their families: group, individual, family, and combination interventions.
- The most frequent types of activities are art, puppets, writing, storytelling, and games.
- Intervention activities are most useful when they are designed to meet the needs of bereaved children (see Chapter 9).

---

[1]For those looking for additional activities to use with bereaved children, I recommend "Waving Goodbye: An Activities Manual for Children in Grief" (1995). Available from the Dougy Center, P. O. Box 86852, Portland, OR 97286.

Epilogue

In the Child Bereavement Study we asked children to tell us what counsel that they would give to other children who are experiencing the death of a parent. Here are some of their responses. In the end it is their wisdom, born of experience, that is the best "counseling" for all of us.

- "Don't ask them a lot of personal questions that make them feel uncomfortable about death," said an 11-year-old girl who lost her mother.
- Her 15-year-old sister told us, "You have to deal with it in your own way. If anything is bothering you, you should say something."
- "Don't try and forget him. If you get another father, keep remembering your real father. Don't give up on things. Don't use your father's death as an excuse," advised an 8-year-old boy.
- "It is important not to give up on your religion. Really, it's the only thing that's been helping me through this. If it wasn't for that, I'm sure I'd just give up on everything," reported a teenage boy who lost his father.
- "It's going to happen sooner or later. Now you won't have to go through it again," was the wisdom of a 9-year-old girl whose father died.
- "Make a bereaved kid feel safe, that nothing is going to happen to them. Don't let them feel guilt; be sure their self-confidence is high," said a 14-year-old boy after his father died.

- "If another kid was in my situation, I'd try to console him. I'd go over to his house and make him talk, go to the wake. I wouldn't give him any advice. I'd try to be quiet," shared a 15-year-old boy who lost his mother.

- "It's hard to live without your father, but it's not like you'll never make it without him, 'cause you'll still live even though he's not alive," said an 11-year-old girl.

- "You don't have to say goodbye; say, 'See you later.' You always think about them but you do get over it," was the hopeful counsel of an 11-year-old girl.

- A young teenage boy offered this advice after his father died: "Just listen to what your parent has to say and don't get offended."

- "Try to understand that individuals have individual problems, not everyone deals with things the same way," said a 13-year-old boy whose father died.

- "Don't be scared. They don't come back and hurt you if you are a little kid," advised a 10-year-old girl who lost her father.

- And, finally, a poignant comment from a 12-year-old boy 2 years after his fathers death: "It is a struggle, but you can survive it. It gets easier as memories come in and the grief goes out."

Project Assessment Instruments

The following are descriptions of the assessment instruments used in the Child Bereavement Study. Some were used in an assessment of the children; others were used to assess the surviving parent and/or the family.

CHILD BEHAVIOR CHECKLIST/4–18
(CBCL; Achenbach, 1991;
Achenbach & Edelbrock, 1983)

Each child's social and emotional behavior was assessed using the CBCL, which consists of 118 behavior problem items rated by parents as "not true," "somewhat or sometimes true," or "very true or often true" of their child. Normalized T scores based on samples of clinical and nonclinical children are available for both the eight narrow-band syndrome scales and the three broad-band scales (total, internalizing, externalizing).

The 1991 version of the CBCL identifies eight behavioral syndromes that can be applied to all children. These syndromes are normed for each of four age–gender quadrants (boys 6–11, boys 12–18, girls 6–11, girls 12–18). These eight scales were determined by factor analysis and utilize 89 of the items from the total 118 items on the CBCL. The eight scales include social withdrawal; somatic complaints; anxiety–depression; social, thought, and attention problems; and delinquent and aggressive behavior.

In addition to the eight narrow-band behavioral syndromes,

there are three broad-band scales. The first, the Total Behavior Problem score, is based on all the items and reflects overall severity of dysfunction. The two other broad-band scales are the internalizing and externalizing scales. These are based on selected syndrome scales and reflect inward-directed (withdrawn behavior, somatic complaints, and anxiety–depression) and outward-directed (aggression and delinquency) problems, respectively.

PERCEIVED COMPETENCE SCALE
FOR CHILDREN
(Harter, 1979, 1985)

Six areas of perceived competence were assessed using this self-report scale: (1) scholastic competence, (2) social competence, (3) athletic competence, (4) physical appearance, (5) behavioral conduct, and (6) global self-worth. The test consists of 28 pairs of statements describing two opposite ends of a specific behavior. Children select the place on the continuum that is "true" or "sort of true" for themselves. Internal consistency values range from .73 to .83.

LOCUS OF CONTROL SCALE FOR CHILDREN
(Nowicki & Strickland, 1973)

This 40-item paper-and-pencil test measures generalized expectancies for internal versus external control of reinforcement among children. It has been used with children from the third grade through college and norms are available for various age groups in that range. The scale has both internal and temporal consistency.

SMILANSKY DEATH QUESTIONNAIRE
(Smilansky, 1987)

This instrument assesses five concepts children have about death: (1) irreversibility, (2) finality, (3) causality, (4) inevitability, and (5) old age. Interrater reliability correlations range from .93 to .97. Equal weight is given to each of the five concepts with a possible score of 15 (0–3 for each concept). The test has construct validity. A test–retest score of .84 was obtained from a random sample of children. Internal reliability was examined by means of Cronbach's alpha based on the correlation between the individual items and the total conceptualization of death. A correlation of .77 was found with all items contributing positively.

FAMILY ADAPTABILITY
AND COHESION EVALUATION SCALES
(FACES-III; Olson et al., 1985)

This 20-item scale is used to measure Family Cohesion (the emotional bonding that family members have toward one another) and Family Adaptability (the ability of a family to change its power structure, role relationships, and relationship rules in response to situational and developmental stress).

Each scale represents a continuum of family functioning. The cohesion scale ranges from extremely low cohesion (disengaged) to moderate levels (separated, connected) to extremely high cohesion (enmeshed). Adaptability ranges from extremely low adaptability (rigid) to moderate levels (structured, flexible) to extremely high adaptability (chaotic). The moderate levels are assumed to be more functional than the extreme levels on each scale.

Internal consistency estimates (alpha) are .87 for family cohesion and .78 for family adaptability. In the normative sample of families, 51% scored in the rigid or structured ranges, 33% scored in the flexible range, and 16% scored in the chaotic range.

FACES-III has discriminated between functional and dysfunctional families in several samples and is considered to be one of the best instruments to assess families on a systems level. Although Olson and his colleagues originally hypothesized a curvilinear relationship between the FACES scales and adjustment, recent findings indicate that the relationship might be linear in samples of nonproblem families (Olson, 1986).

FAMILY INVENTORY OF LIFE EVENTS
(FILE; McCubbin et al., 1979)

The FILE is a checklist of stressors that a family might experience. It was developed for the differential assessment of changes experienced by a family within a given time period. We adapted the list of 72 stressors to apply to the single-parent bereaved family. The items have face validity and are grouped into topical areas such as strains around legal and financial losses, sexuality, school, substance abuse, and family responsibilities.

FAMILY CRISIS ORIENTED
PERSONAL EVALUATION SCALES
(F-COPES; McCubbin et al., 1982)

F-COPES is a measure of family coping responses to various problems and difficulties. It is composed of six different scales. The scale was developed to assess two dimensions of family interaction: (1) internal family strategies (ways families use resources residing within the nuclear system, such as the ability to reframe family problems) and (2) external family strategies (the family's ability to acquire resources outside the nuclear system, such as the resources of religion, friends, extended family, and community). The 29-item Likert-type scale identifies eight major coping approaches: (1) confidence in family problem solving, (2) reframing family problems, (3) family passivity, (4) religious resources, (5) extended family, (6) friends, (7) neighbors, and (8) community resources. The test has adequate construct validity. The scales have alpha reliabilities ranging from .64 to .87, and acceptable test–retest reliabilities from .49 to .85

CENTER FOR EPIDEMIOLOGICAL
STUDIES—DEPRESSION SCALE
(CES-D; Radloff, 1977)

Depressive symptomatology was measured with the CES-D. The CES-D was developed for use in studies of the epidemiology of depressive symptomatology in the general population. This 20-item scale assesses how often depressive symptoms had occurred during the past week and includes a report of general dysphoric mood, lack of positive mood, and vegetative symptoms. Radloff and her colleagues have reviewed the literature using the CES-D and have found it to have adequate reliability and criterion-related validity using self-report and clinician-rated variables in both psychiatric and large community populations (Radloff & Teri, 1986).

IMPACT OF EVENTS SCALE
(IES; Zilberg et al. 1982)

We also administered the IES to the surviving parents. This self-report instrument assesses the essential characteristics associated with stress disorders. The IES is a 15-item two-dimensional scale measuring intrusive thoughts and avoidant thinking or denial patterns of the traumatic event.

Screening Instrument
and Instrument Scoring

INSTRUMENT DEVELOPMENT

To develop a screening instrument, we randomly divided the bereaved children into two groups, a screening sample and a cross-validation sample. Our criterion variable was the child's risk score at the 1- and 2-year assessments. We had originally planned to construct two screening instruments—one to predict risk at 1 year and the other to predict risk at 2 years. However, because of the limited number of children in the risk group at any one time point, it seemed advisable to combine the groups to increase sample size. If the child was in the risk group at either the first and/or second anniversaries, he or she was placed into the high-risk group. If not, the child was placed into the low-risk group. This approach also makes good clinical sense. Even if a child was only in the risk group at the second anniversary, very early intervention could possibly prevent a later adaptation.

We selected six prediction variables (see "Instrument Scoring") that had high correlation with our criterion variable and low intercorrelation with each other. The following variables came from Time data gathered 4 months after the death:

1. Surviving parent's age
2. Number of children in family under age 12
3. Parent's stress scale score

4. Parent's coping scale score
5. Parent's depression score (CES-D)
6. The child's total score on the CBCL.

We used a unit-weighted approach for each variable, assigning a value of 1 to scores on the variable exceeding 0.5 standard deviation above the mean for that variable and a value of 0 for the rest. We chose a unit-weighted approach rather than using multiple regression Beta coefficients because the results of this approach are more applicable to other groups (Worden, 1984).

A child's total risk score was the sum of the 6 unit-weighted scores (0 to 6). These total risk scores correlated .42 (point biserial) with the criterion variable for the screening sample ($N = 56$) and .43 for the cross-validation sample ($N = 57$). Using a cutoff score of 3 or higher, risk scores correctly predicted 82% on the screening sample, 81% on the cross-validation sample, and 81% on the total group of children. Of the 19% misses, false negatives accounted for one-quarter, while three-quarters were false positives. It should be noted that all of the predictors came from information supplied by the parent rather than data gathered from the children themselves. Not only did these variables prove to be the best predictors, but we believed that a screening instrument would be easier to administer to a surviving parent than to the children themselves. This instrument should only be used with parentally bereaved children between ages 6 and 18, and completed by the surviving parent within 6 months after death.

SCREENING INSTRUMENT

Parent's name: _____ Date: _____

1. Parent's age: _____

2. Number of children in family under age 12: _____

3. Stress: According to the scale below, how stressful has the past few months been for you? (circle one)

   Not stressful   1   2   3   4   5   6   7   8   Very stressful

4. Coping: At this point in time, how well do you feel you are coping with your loss? (circle one)

   Not at all   1   2   3   4   5   6   7   8   Very well

5. CES-D: Below is a list of ways you might have felt or behaved. Please tell us how often you have felt this way during the past week: (circle a number for each item)

		Rarely or never	1–2 days	3–4 days	5–7 days
a.	I was bothered by things that usually don't bother me . . .	0	1	2	3
b.	I did not feel like eating; my appetite was poor . . .	0	1	2	3
c.	I felt that I could not shake off the blues even with help from my family or friends . . .	0	1	2	3
d.	I felt that I was just as good as other people . . .	0	1	2	3
e.	I had trouble keeping my mind on what I was doing . . .	0	1	2	3
f.	I felt depressed . . .	0	1	2	3

g.	I felt that everything I did was an effort . . .	0	1	2	3
h.	I felt hopeful about the future . . .	0	1	2	3
i.	I thought my life had been a failure . . .	0	1	2	3
j.	I felt fearful . . .	0	1	2	3
k.	My sleep was restless . . .	0	1	2	3
l.	I was happy . . .	0	1	2	3
m.	I talked less than usual . . .	0	1	2	3
n.	I felt lonely . . .	0	1	2	3
o.	People were unfriendly . . .	0	1	2	3
p.	I enjoyed life . . .	0	1	2	3
q.	I had crying spells . . .	0	1	2	3
r.	I felt sad . . .	0	1	2	3
s.	I felt that people disliked me . . .	0	1	2	3
t.	I could not get "going" . . .	0	1	2	3

6. CBCL: Please fill out a Child Behavior Checklist for each of your children.

INSTRUMENT SCORING

Here is a way to score the information obtained on the screening instrument:

1. Age of parent: _____
    if 39 or older, code = 0
    if 38 or younger, code = 1

2. Number of children in family under 12 years of age: _____
    if 1 or 2, code = 0
    if 3 or more, code = 1

3. Stress scale score: _____
    if 1–7, code = 0
    if 8, code = 1

4. Coping scale score: _____
    if 1–5, code = 0
    if 6–8, code = 1

5. Parent's CES-D score:[1]   _____
    if 0–24, code = 0
    if 25 or greater, code = 1

6. Child's CBCL total score: _____
    if 55 or lower, code = 0
    if 56 or higher, code = 1

TOTAL SCREENING SCORE: _____
(Add scores 1 through 6)

If the Total Screening Score equals 0–2, the child is not expected to be at risk 1 or 2 years after the loss. If the Total Screening Score equals 3–6, the child is projected to be in the risk group, and early intervention should be considered.

[1]On the CES-D, use reverse scoring for items d, h, l, and p.

Suggested Readings

GENERAL REFERENCES
ON CHILDREN AND BEREAVEMENT

Altschul, S., & Pollock, G. H. (Eds.). (1988). *Childhood bereavement and its aftermath*. New York: International Universities Press.

Anthony, S. (1971). *The discovery of death in childhood and after.* London: Penguin.

Arthur, B., & Kemme, M. (1964). Bereavement in childhood. *Journal of Child Psychology and Psychiatry, 5,* 37–49.

Baker, J. E., Sedney, M. A., & Gross, E. (1992). Psychological tasks for bereaved children. *American Journal of Orthopsychiatry, 62,* 105–116.

Beard, P. (1989). A bereaved child. *Nursing Times, 85,* 59–61.

Becker, D., & Margolin, F. (1967). How surviving parents handled their young children's adaptation to the crisis of loss. *American Journal of Orthopsychiatry, 37,* 753–757.

Bentovim, A. (1986). Bereaved children. *British Medical Journal, 292,* 1482.

Berden, G., Althous, M., & Verhulst, F. (1990). Major life events and changes in the behavioral functioning of children. *Journal of Clinical Psychology and Psychiatry, 31,* 949–959.

Black, D. (1974). What happens to bereaved children? *Proceedings of the Royal Society of Medicine, 69,* 38–40.

Black, D. (1978). The bereaved child. *Journal of Child Psychology and Psychiatry, 19,* 287–292.

Bowlby, J. (1960). Grief and mourning in infancy and early childhood. *Psychoanalytic Study of the Child, 15,* 9–52.

Bowlby, J. (1961). Childhood mourning and its implications for psychiatry. *American Journal of Psychiatry, 118,* 481–498.

Cheifetz, P. N., Stavrakakis, G., & Lester, E. P. (1989). Studies of the affective state in bereaved children. *Canadian Journal of Psychiatry, 34*(7), 688–692.

Chetnik, M. (1970). The impact of object loss on a six year old. *Journal of the American Academy of Child Psychiatry, 9,* 624–643

Fitzgerald, H. (1992). *The grieving child: A parent's guide.* New York: Simon & Schuster.

Fleming, S. J. (1985). Children's grief. In C. A. Corr & D. M. Corr (Eds.), *Hospice approaches to pediatric care* (pp. 197–218). New York: Springer.

Fox, S. (1985). Children's aniversary reactions to the death of a family member. *Omega, 15,* 291–305.

Freeman, E. M. (1984). Loss and grief in children: Implications for school social workers. *Social Work Education, 6,* 241–258.

Furman, E. (1983). Studies in childhood bereavement. *Canadian Journal of Psychiatry, 28,* 241–247.

Furman, R. (1964). Death and the young child: Some preliminary considerations. *Psychoanalytic Study of the Child, 19,* 321–333.

Furman, R. A. (1970). The child's reaction to death in the family. In B. Schoenberg & A. Carr (Eds.), *Loss and grief: Psychological management in medical practice* (pp. 70–86). New York: Columbia University Press.

Furman, R. A. (1973). A child's capacity for mourning. In E. Anthony & C. Koupernik (Eds.), *The child and his family.* New York: Wiley.

Hagin, R. S., & Corwin, C. G. (1974). Bereaved children. *Journal of Clinical Child Psychology, 3,* 39–46.

Harrison, S., Davenport, D., & Mc Dermott, J. (1967). Children's reactions to bereavement. *Archives of General Psychiatry, 17,* 593–597.

Kliman, G. (Ed.). (1968). *Psychological emergencies in childhood.* New York: Grune & Stratton.

Kliman, G. (1977). The children. In N. Linzer (Ed.), *Understanding bereavement and grief.* New York: Yeshiva University Press.

Kliman, G. (1989). Facilitation of mourning during childhood. In S. Klagsbrun, G. Kliman, E. Clark, et al. (Eds.), *Preventive psychiatry* (pp. 59–82). Philadelphia: Charles.

Koocher, G. P. (1983). Grief and loss in childhood. In C. E. Walker & M. C. Roberts (Eds.), *Handbook of clinical child psychology.* New York: Wiley.

Lamers, E. P. (1983). Children, school and death. *Alberta Learning Resources Journal, 5,* 6–14.

Lubowe, S. (1989). Prevention in major childhood bereavement. In S. Klagsbrun, G. Kliman, E. Clark, et al. (Eds.), *Preventive psychiatry.* Philadelphia: Charles.

Mahler, M. S. (1961). On sadness and grief in infancy and childhood. *Psychoanalytic Study of the Child, 16,* 332–351.

Munro, A., & Griffiths, A. B. (1969). Some psychiatric non-sequelae of childhood bereavement. *British Journal of Psychiatry, 115,* 305–311.

Parnass, E. (1975). Effects of experiences with loss and death among pre-school children. *Children Today, 4,* 2–7.

Plotkin, D. R. (1983). Children's anniversary reaction following the death of a family member. *Canada's Mental Health, 31,* 13–15.

Rudolph, M. (1978). *Should the children know? Encounters with death in the lives of children.* New York: Schocken.

Saladay, S. A., & Royal, M. E. (1981). Children and death: Guidelines for grief work. *Child Psychiatry and Human Development, 11,* 203–212.

Schowalter, J. et al. (Eds). (1983). *The child and death.* New York: Columbia University Press.

Sekaer, C. (1987). Toward a definition of "childhood mourning." *American Journal of Psychotherapy, 41,* 201–219.

Sekaer, C., & Katz, S. (1986). On the concept of mourning in childhood: Reactions of a 2½-year-old girl to the death of her father. *Psychoanalytic Study of the Child, 41,* 287–314.

Silverman, P. R., & Silverman, S. M. (1975). Withdrawal in bereaved children. In A. Schoenberg et al. (Eds.), *Bereavement: Its psychological aspects.* New York: Columbia University Press.

Sood, B., Weller, E., Weller, R., et al. (1992). Somatic complaints in grieving children. *Comprehensive Mental Health Care, 2,* 17–25.

Tallmer, M. (1975). Sexual and age factors in childhood bereavement. In A. Schoenberg et al. (Eds.), *Bereavement: Its psychological aspects.* New York: Columbia University Press.

Van Eerdewegh, M. M., Clayton, P. J., & Van Eerdewegh, P. (1985). The bereaved child: Variables influencing early psychopathology. *British Journal of Psychiatry, 14,* 188–194.

Vida, S., & Grizenko, N. (1989). DSM-III-R and the phenomenology of childhood bereavement: A review. *Canadian Journal of Psychiatry, 34*(2), 148–155.

Wass, H., & Corr, C. (Eds.). (1984). *Childhood and death.* New York: Hemisphere.

Wolfenstein, M. (1966). How is mourning possible? *Psychoanalytic Study of the Child, 21,* 93–123.

Wolff, S. (1969). *Bereavement in children under stress.* London: Penguin.

DEATH OF A PARENT

Albert, R. S. (1971). Cognitive development and parental loss among the gifted, the exceptionally gifted and creative. *Psychological Reports, 29,* 19–26.

Berlinsky, E. B., & Biller, H. B. (1982). *Parental death and psychological development*. Lexington, MA: D. C. Heath.

Cain, A. C., & Fast, I. (1966). Children's disturbed reactions to parent suicide. *American Journal of Orthopsychiatry, 5*, 873–880.

Eisenstadt, J. M. (1978, March). Parental loss and genius. *American Psychologist*, 211–223.

Elizur, E., & Kaffman, M. (1982). Children's bereavement reactions following death of the father: II. *Journal of the American Academy of Child Psychiatry, 21*, 474–480.

Elizur, E., & Kaffman, M. (1983). Factors influencing the severity of childhood bereavement reactions. *American Journal of Orthopsychiatry, 53*, 668–676.

Felner, R. D. et al. (1981). Parental death or divorce and the school adjustment of young children. *American Journal of Community Psychology, 9*, 181–191.

Fristad, M., Jedel, R., Weller, R., & Weller, E. (1993). Psychosocial functioning in children after the death of a parent. *American Journal of Psychiatry, 150*, 511–513.

Furman, E. (1974). *A child's parent dies: Studies in childhood bereavement*. New Haven, CT: Yale University Press.

Furman, E. (1986). On trauma: When is the death of a parent traumatic? *Psychoanalytic Study of the Child, 41*, 191–208.

Gregory, I. (1965). Anterospective data following childhood loss of a parent. *Archives of General Psychiatry, 13*, 110–120.

Grossberg, S. H., & Crandall, L. (1978). Father loss and father absence in pre-school children. *Clinical Social Work Journal, 6*, 123–134.

Hepworth, J., Ryder R., & Dreyer, A. (1984). The effects of parental loss on the formation of intimate relationships. *Journal of Marital and Family Therapy, 10*, 73–82.

Johnson, P. A. (1982). After a child's parent has died. *Child Psychiatry and Human Development, 12*, 160–170.

Johnson, P. A., & Rosenblatt, P. C. (1981). Grief following childood loss of a parent. *American Journal of Psychotherapy, 35*, 419–425.

Kaffman, M., & Elizur, E. (1979). Children's bereavement reactions following death of the father. *International Journal of Family Therapy, 1*, 203–229.

Kaffman, M., & Elizur, E. (1983). Bereavement responses of kibbutz and non-kibbutz children following the death of the father. *Journal of Child Psychology and Psychiatry, 24*, 435–442.

Kranzler, E. M., Shaffer, D., Wasserman, G., et al. (1990). Early childhood bereavement. *Journal of the American Academy of Child and Adolescent Psychiatry, 29*, 513–520.

Krementz, J. (1991). *How it feels when a parent dies.* New York: Knopf.

Laajus, S. (1984). Parental losses. *Acta Psychiatrica Scandinavica, 69,* 1–12.

Leaverton, D. R. et al. (1980). Parental loss antecedent to childhood Diabetes Mellitus. *Journal of the American Academy of Child Psychiatry, 19,* 678–688.

LeShan, E. (1976). *Learning to say good-bye when a parent dies.* New York: Macmillan.

Lifshitz, M. (1976). Long range effects of father's loss: The cognitive complexity of bereaved children and their social adjustment. *British Journal of Medical Psychology, 49,* 189–197.

Lifshitz, M., Berman, D., Galili, A., et al. (1977). Bereaved children: The effect of mother's perceptions and social system on their short-range adjustment. *Journal of the American Academy of Child Psychiatry, 16,* 272–284.

Miller, J. B. M. (1971). Children's reactions to the death of a parent: A review of psychoanylitic literature. *Journal of the American Psychoanalytic Association, 19,* 697–719.

Mireault, G. C., & Bond, L. A. (1992). Parental death in childhood: Perceived vulnerability, and adult depression and anxiety. *American Journal of Orthopsychiatry, 62,* 517–524.

Palmer, A. J. (1984). Tom Sawyer: Early parental loss. *Bulletin of the Menninger Clinic, 48,* 155–169.

Polombo, J. (1981). Parent loss and childhood bereavement: Some theoretical considerations. *Clinical Social Work, 9,* 3–33.

Raphael, B. (1982). The young child and the death of a parent. In C. M. Parkes & J. Stevenson-Hinde (Eds.), *The place of attachment in human behavior.* New York: Basic Books.

Rutter, M. (1966). *Children of sick parents.* London: Oxford University Press.

Sandler, I., Gersten, J., Reynolds, K., et al. (1988). Using theory and data to plan support interventions. In B. Gottlieb (Ed.), *Marshalling social support.* Newbury Park, CA: Sage.

Silverman, S. M. (1974). Parental loss and scientists. *Science Studies, 4,* 259–264.

Strength, J. M. (1991). Factors influencing the mother–child relationship following the death of the father. *Dissertation Abstracts International, 52,* 3310B.

Van Eerdewegh, M., Bieri, M., Parilla, R. H., & Clayton, P. J. (1982). The bereaved child. *British Journal of Psychiatry, 140,* 23–29.

Weller, R. A., Weller, E. B., Fristad, M. A., & Bowes, J. M. (1991). Depression in recently bereaved prepubertal children. *American Journal of Psychiatry, 148,* 1536–1540.

Wolfenstein, M. (1965). Death of a parent and death of a president. In M. Wolfenstein & G. Kliman G. (Eds.), *Children and death of a president.* New York: Doubleday.

BEREAVED ADOLESCENTS

Balk, D. E. (1996). Models for understanding adolescent coping with bereavement. *Death Studies, 20,* 367–387.

Bemporad, J. R., Ratey, J., & Hallowell, E. M. (1986). Loss and depression in young adults. *Journal of the American Academy of Psychoanalysis, 14,* 167–179.

Berman, H., Cragg, C. E., & Kuenzig, L. (1988). Having a parent die of cancer: Adolescents' reactions. *Oncology Nursing Forum, 15,* 159–163.

Bright, P. D. (1987). Adolescent pregnancy and loss. *Maternal Child Nursing Journal, 16,* 1–12.

Corr, C. A., & Balk, D. E. (Eds.). (1996). *Handbook of adolescence and bereavement.* New York: Springer.

Dietrich, D. R. (1984). Psychological health of young adults who experienced early parental death: MMPI trends. *Journal of Clinical Psychology, 40,* 901–908.

Freudenberger, H. J., & Gallagher, K. M. (1995). Emotional consequences of loss four our adolescents. *Psychotherapy, 32,* 150–153.

Garber, B. (1983). Some thoughts on normal adolescents who lost a parent by death. *Journal of Youth and Adolescents, 12,* 175–182.

Garber, B. (1985). Mourning in adolescence: Normal and pathological. *Adolescent Psychiatry, 12,* 371–387.

Glass, J. C. (1990). Death, loss, and grief in high school students. *High School Journal, 73,* 154–160.

Gravelle, K., & Haskins, C. (1989). *Teenagers face to face with bereavement.* New York: Messner.

Gray, R. E. (1987a). The role of the surviving parent in the adaptation of bereaved adolescents. *Journal of Palliative Care, 3,* 30–34.

Gray, R. E. (1987b). Adolescent response to the death of a parent. *Journal of Youth and Adolescence, 16,* 511–525.

Gray, R. E. (1989). Adolescents' perceptions of social support after the death of a parent. *Journal of Psychosocial Oncology, 7*(3), 127–144.

Harris, E. S. (1991). Adolescent bereavement following the death of a parent: An exploratory study. *Child Psychiatry and Human Development, 2,* 267–281.

Hetherington, M. (1972). Effects of father absence on personality development in adolescent daughters. *Developmental Psychology, 7,* 313–326.

Kaltreider, N. B., Becker, J., & Horowitz, M. J. (1984). Relationship testing after the loss of a parent. *American Journal of Psychiatry, 141,* 243–246.

Kaltreider, N., & Mendelson, S. (1985). Clinical evaluation of grief after parental death. *Psychotherapy, 22,* 224–230.

Meshot, C. M., & Leitner, L. M. (1992). Adolescent mourning and parental death. *Omega, 26,* 287–299.

Meshot, C. M., & Leitner, L. M. (1993). Death threat, parental loss, and interpersonal style. *Death Studies, 17,* 319–332.

Murphy, P. A. (1986). Parental death in childhood and loneliness in young adults. *Omega, 17,* 219–228.

Podell, C. (1989). Adolescent mourning: The sudden death of a peer. *Clinical Social Work Journal, 17*(1), 64–78.

Seligman, R., Gleser, G., & Raugh, J. (1974). The effects of earlier parental loss in adolescence. *Archives of General Psychiatry, 31,* 475–479.

Smith, G. R. et al. (1988). Panic and nausea instead of grief in an adolescent. *Journal of the American Academy of Child and Adolscent Psychiatry, 27,* 509–513.

Sugar, M. (1968). Normal adolescent mourning. *American Journal of Psychotherapy, 22,* 258–269.

Werner, A., & Jones, M. (1979). Parent loss in college students. *Journal of the American College Health Association, 27,* 253–255.

CHILDREN AND DIVORCE

Brown, J., Eichenberger, S., Portes, P., et al. (1992). Family functioning factors associated with the adjustment of children of divorce. *Journal of Divorce and Remarriage, 17,* 81–95.

Cherlin, A. J. et al. (1991). Longitudinal studies of effects of divorce on children in Great Britain and the United States. *Science, 252,* 1386–1389.

Copeland, A. P. (1985). Individual differences in children's reactions to divorce. *Journal of Clinical Child Psychology, 14,* 11–19.

Doka, K. J. (1986). Loss upon loss: The impact of death after divorce. *Death Studies, 10,* 441–450.

Fogas, B., Wolchik, S., Braver, S., et al. (1992). Locus of control as a mediator of negative divorce-related events and adjustment problems in children. *American Journal of Orthopsychiatry, 62,* 589–598.

Francke, L. B. (1983). *Growing up divorced.* New York: Fawcett.

Healy, J. M., Stewart, A. J., & Copeland, A. P. (1993). The role of self-blame in children's adjustment to parental separation. *Personality and Social Psychology Bulletin, 19,* 279–289.

Hetherington, E. M. (1979). Divorce: A child's perspective. *American Psychologist, 43.*

Hetherington, E. M. (1987). Family relations six years after divorce. In R. Hinde & J. Stevenson (Eds.), *Relations six years after divorce.* New York: Guilford Press.

Hetherington, E. M. (1993). An overview of the Virginia longitudinal study of divorce and remarriage with a focus on early adolescence. *Journal of Family Psychology, 7,* 39–56.

Hetherington, E. M., & Deur, J. (1971). The effects of father absence on child development. *Young Children, 26,* 233–248.

Kalter, N., Kloner, A., Schreier, S., et al. (1989). Predictors of children's postdivorce adjustment. *American Journal of Orthopsychiatry, 59,* 605–618.

Kurdek, L. A. (1991). Differences in ratings of children's adjustment by married mothers. *Journal of Applied Developmental Psychology, 12,* 289.

Mishne, J. M. (1984). Trauma of parent loss through divorce, death and illness. *Child and Adolescent Social Work Journal, 1,* 74–88.

Portes, P. R. et al. (1992). Family functions and children's post divorce adjustment. *American Journal of Orthopsychiatry, 62,* 613–617.

Sandler, I., Wolchik, S., Braver, S., et al. (1991). Stability and quality of life events and psychological symptomatology in children of divorce. *American Journal of Community Psychology, 19,* 501–520.

Stolberg, A. L., & Garrison, K. M. (1985). Evaluating a primary prevention program for children of divorce. *American Journal of Community Psychology, 13,* 111–124.

Tessman, L. H. (1978). *Children of parting parents.* New York: Jason Aronson.

Tschann, J., Johnston, J., Kline, M., et al. (1990). Conflict, loss, change, and parent–child relationships: Predicting children's adjustment during divorce. *Journal of Divorce, 13,* 1–22.

Wakerman, E. (1984). *Father loss: Daughters discuss the man that got away.* New York: Doubleday.

Wallerstein, J. S. (1983). Children of divorce: The psychological tasks of the child. *American Journal of Orthopsychiatry, 53,* 230–243.

Wallerstein, J. S. (1991). The long-term effects of divorce on children: A review. *Journal of the American Academy of Child and Adolescent Psychiatry, 30.*

Wallerstein, J. S., & Blakeslee, S. (1989). *Second chances: Men, women, and children a decade after divorce.* New York: Ticknor & Fields.

Wallerstein, J. S., & Kelly, J. B. (1980). *Surviving the breakup: How children and parents cope with divorce.* New York: Basic Books.

FAMILIES AND GRIEF

Agee, J. (1957). *A death in the family.* New York: Bantam.

Archer, D. N., & Smith, A. C. (1988). Sorrow has many faces: Helping families cope with grief. *Nursing, 18,* 43–45.

Bengesser, G. (1988). Postvention for bereaved family members: Some therapeutic possibilities. *Crisis, 9*(1), 45–48.

Black, D. (1984). Sundered families: The effect of loss of a parent. *Adoption and Fostering, 8,* 34–43.

Black, D., & Urbanowicz, M. A. (1987). Family intervention with bereaved children. *Journal of Child Psychology and Psychiatry, 28,* 467–476.

Bowlby-West, L. (1983). The impact of death on the family system. *Journal of Family Therapy, 5,* 279–294.

Crase, D. R., & Crase, D. (1989). Single-child families and death. *Childhood Education, 65,* 153–156.

Dailey, A. A. (1988). About our children. Approaching grief for parents and siblings. *American Journal of Hospice Care, 5,* 10–12.

Davies, B., Spinetta, J., Martinson, I., et al. (1986). Manifestations of levels of functioning in grieving families. *Journal of Family Issues, 7,* 297–313.

Detmer, C. M., & Lamberti, J. W. (1991). Family grief. *Death Studies, 15,* 363–374.

Fulmer, R. H. (1987). Special problems of mourning in low-income single-parent families. *Family Therapy Collective, 23,* 19–37.

Gelcer, E. (1983). Mourning is a family affair. *Family Process, 22,* 501–516.

Gelcer, E. (1986). Dealing with loss in the family context. *Journal of Family Issues, 7,* 315–335.

Goldberg, S. B. (1973). Family tasks and reactions in the crisis of death. *Social Casework, 54,* 398–405.

Greaves, C. C. (1983). Death in the family: A multifamily therapy approach. *International Journal of Family Psychiatry, 4,* 247–259.

Jensen, G. D., & Wallace, J. G. (1967). Family mourning process. *Family Process, 6,* 56–66.

Kuhn, J. S. (1977). Realignment of emotional forces following loss. *Family, 5,* 19–24.

Lieberman, M. A. (1989). All family losses are not equal. *Journal of Family Psychology, 2*(3), 368–372.

McClowry, S. G., Davies, E. B., May, E. J., et al. (1987). The empty space phenomenon: The process of grief in the bereaved family. *Death Studies, 11,* 361–374.

Morgan, L. A. (1984). Changes in family interaction following widowhood. *Journal of Marriage and the Family, 46,* 323–331.

Owen, G., Fulton, R., & Markusen, E. (1982–1983). Death at a distance: A study of family survivors. *Omega, 13,* 191–225.

Paul, N., & Grosser, G. H. (1965). Operational mourning and its role in conjoint family therapy. *Community Mental Health Journal, 1,* 339–345.

Pietropinto, A. (1985). Coping with death in the family. *Medical Aspects of Human Sexuality, 19,* 76–82.

Pincus, L. (1972). *Death and the family.* New York: Pantheon.

Reilly, D. M. (1978). Death propensity, dying, and bereavement: A family systems perspective. *Family Therapy, 5,* 35–55.

Schneiderman, G. (1979). *Coping with death in the family.* Oakville, Canada: Chimo.

Silverman, P. R. (1975). The widow's view of her dependent children. *Omega, 6,* 3–19.

Silverman, S. M., & Silverman, P. R. (1979). Parent–child communication in widowed families. *American Journal of Psychotherapy, 33,* 428–441.

Vess, J., Moreland, J., & Schwebel, A. (1985–1986). Understanding family role reallocation following a death: A theoretical framework. *Omega, 16,* 115–128.

Walsh, F., & McGoldrick, M. (1991). *Living beyond loss: Death in the family.* New York: Norton.

Weber, J. A., & Fournier, D. G. (1985). Family support and a child's adjustment to death. *Family Relations, 34,* 43–49.

Wedemeyer, N. V. (1986). Death is part of family life. *Journal of Family Issues, 7,* 235–236.

Wessel, M. A. (1975). A death in the family: The impact on children. *Journal of the American Medical Association, 234,* 865–866.

Worden, J. W., & Silverman, P. R. (1993). Grief and depression in newly widowed parents with school-age children. *Omega, 27*(3), 251–260.

INTERVENTION WITH BEREAVED CHILDREN

Adams-Greenly, M. (1984). Helping children communicate about serious illness and death. *Journal of Psychosocial Oncology, 2,* 61–73.

Bertman, S. (1983). Helping children cope with death. In T. T. Frantz & J. C. Hansen (Eds.), *Death in the family.* Rockville, MD: Aspen.

Carey, L. (1990). Sandplay therapy with a troubled child. *Arts in Psychotherapy, 17,* 197–209.

Carter, P. (1986). School nursing: Helping children to grieve. *Community Outlook, 13,* 16–17.

Christ, G., Siegel, K., Mesagno, F., et al. (1991). A preventive intervention

Bendiksen, R., & Fulton, R. (1975). Childhood bereavement and later disorders. *Omega, 6,* 45–60.

Birtchnell, J. (1970a). Depression in relation to early and recent parent death. *British Journal of Psychiatry, 116,* 299–305.

Birtchnell, J. (1970b). Early parent death and mental health. *British Journal of Psychiatry, 116,* 281–298.

Birtchnell, J. (1972). Early parent death and psychiatric diagnosis. *Social Psychiatry, 7,* 202–210.

Birtchnell, J. (1980). Women whose mothers died in childhood: An outcome study. *Psychological Medicine, 10,* 699–713.

Bowlby, J. (1963). Pathological mourning and childhood mourning. *Journal American Psychoanalytic Association, 11,* 500–541

Breier, A., Kelso, J., Kirwin, P., et al. (1988). Early parental loss and development of adult psychopathology. *Archives of General Psychiatry, 45,* 987–993.

Brown, F., & Epps, P. (1966). Childhood bereavement and subsequent crime. *British Journal of Psychiatry, 112,* 1043–1048.

Brown, G. W., & Harris, T. O. (1986). Establishing causal links. In H. Katsching (Ed.), *Life events and psychiatric disorders: Controversal issues* (pp. 107–187). Cambridge: Cambridge University Press.

Brown, G. W., Harris, T. O., & Bifulco, A. (1986). Long term effects of early loss of parent. In M. Rutter, C. E. Izard, & P. Read (Eds.), *Depression in young people.* New York: Guilford Press.

Brown, G., Harris, L., & Copeland, J. (1977). Depression and loss. *British Journal of Psychiatry, 130,* 1–18.

Coryell, W., Noyes, R., & Clancy, J. (1983). Panic disorder and primary unipolar depression. *Journal Affective Disorders, 5,* 311–317.

Crook, T., & Raskin, A. (1975). Association of childhood parental loss with attempted suicide and depression. *Journal of Consulting and Clinical Psychology, 43,* 277.

Dennehy, C. (1966). Childhood bereavement and psychiatric illness. *British Journal of Psychiatry, 112,* 1049–1069.

Deutsch, H. (1937). Absence of grief. *Psychoanalytic Quarterly, 6,* 12–22.

Edelman, H. (1994). *Motherless daughters: The legacy of loss.* New York: Dell.

Faravelli, C., Webb, T., Ambonetti, A., et al. (1985). Prevalence of traumatic early life events in 31 agoraphobic patients with panic attacks. *American Journal of Psychiatry, 142,* 1493–1494.

Finkelstein, H. (1988). The long-term effects of early parent death: A review. *Journal of Clinical Psychology, 44,* 3–9.

Harris, M. (1995). *The loss that is forever: The lifelong impact of the early death of a mother or father.* New York: Dutton

Harris, T., Brown, G. W., & Bifulco, A. (1986). Loss of parent in childhood and adult psychiatric disorders: The role of lack of adequate parental care. *Psychological Medicine, 16,* 641–659.

Kendler, K. S., Neale, M. C., Kessler, R. C., et al. (1992). Childhood parental loss and adult psychopathology in women: A twin study perspective. *Archives of General Psychiatry, 49,* 109–116.

Klerman, G., & Weissman, M. (1986). The interpersonal approach to understanding depression. In T. Millon & G. Klerman (Eds.), *Contemporary directions in psychopathology.* New York: Guilford Press.

Lloyd, C. (1980). Life events and depressive disorder reviewed. *Archives of General Psychiatry, 37,* 529–535.

Markusen, E., & Fulton, R. (1971). Childhood bereavement and behavioral disorders: A critical review. *Omega, 2,* 107–117.

Raskin, M., Peeke, H., Dickman, W., et al. (1982). Panic and generalized anxiety disorders: Developmental antecedents and precipitants. *Archives of General Psychiatry, 39,* 687–689.

Saler, L., & Skolnick, N. (1992). Childhood parental death and depression in adulthood: Roles of surviving parent and family enviornment. *American Journal of Orthopsychiatry, 62,* 504–516.

Silverman, P. R. (1989). The impact of parental death on college-age women. *Psychiatric Clinics of North America, 10,* 387–404.

Tennant, C. (1988). Parental loss in childhood: Its effect in adult life. *Archives of General Psychiatry, 45,* 1045–1049.

Tennant, C., Bebbington, P., & Hurry, J. (1980). Parent death in childhood and risk of adult depressive disorders: A review. *Psychological Medicine, 10,* 289–299.

Tennant, C., Bebbington, P., & Hurry, J. (1981). Parental loss in childhood: Relationship to adult psychiatric impairment and contact with psychiatric services. *Archives of General Psychiatry, 38,* 309–314.

Torgersen, S. (1986). Childhood and family characteristics in panic and generalized anxiety disorders. *American Journal of Psychiatry, 143,* 630–632.

Tweed, J., Schoenbach, V., George, L., et al. (1989). The effect of childhood parental death and divorce on six-month history of anxiety disorders. *British Journal of Psychiatry, 154,* 823–828.

Watt, N. F., & Nicholi, A. (1979). Early death of a parent as an etiological factor in schizophrenia. *American Journal of Orthopsychiatry, 49,* 465–473.

Wilson, I. C., Altop, L., & Buffaloe, W. J. (1967). Parental bereavement in childhood: MMPI profiles in a depressed population. *British Journal of Psychiatry, 113,* 761–764.

SIBLING DEATHS

Balk, D. (1983a). Effects of sibling deaths on teenagers. *Journal of School Health, 53,* 14–18.

Balk, D. E. (1983b). Adolescents' grief reactions and self-concept perceptions following sibling death. *Journal of Youth and Adolescence, 12,* 137–161.

Balk, D. E. (1990a). The self-concepts of bereaved adolescents: Sibling death and its aftermath. *Journal of Adolescent Research, 5*(1), 112–132.

Balk, D. E. (1990b). Adolescent reactions to sibling death: Perceptions of mothers, fathers, and teenagers. *Nursing Research, 39,* 103–105.

Birenbaum, L. K., Robinson, M., Phillips, D., et al. (1989). The response of children to the dying and death of a sibling. *Omega, 20,* 213–228.

Blinder, B. (1972). Sibling death in childhood. *Child Psychiatry and Human Development, 2,* 169–175.

Burns, E. A., House, J. D., & Ankenbauer, M. R. (1986). Sibling grief in reaction to sudden death syndrome. *Pediatrics, 78,* 485–487.

Cain, A. C., Fast, I., & Erickson, M. E. (1964). Children's disturbed reactions to the death of a sibling. *American Journal of Orthopsychiatry, 34,* 741–752.

Davies, B. (1988a). The family environment in bereaved families and its relationship to surviving sibling behavior. *Children's Health Care, 17,* 22–32.

Davies, B. (1988b). Shared life space and sibling bereavement responses. *Cancer Nursing, 11,* 339–347.

Davies, B. (1991). Long-term outcomes of adolescent sibling bereavement. *Journal of Adolescent Research, 6,* 83–96.

Demi, A., & Gilbert, C. (1987). Relationship of parental grief to sibling grief. *Archives of Psychiatric Nursing, 6,* 385–391.

Fanos, J. H., & Nickerson, B. G. (1991). Long-term effects of sibling death during adolescence. *Journal of Adolescent Research, 6,* 70–82.

Feinberg, D. (1970). Preventive therapy with siblings of a dying child. *Journal of the American Academy of Child Psychiatry, 9,* 644–668.

Heiney, S. P. (1991). Sibling grief: A case report. *Archives of Psychiatric Nursing, 5,* 121–127.

Hogan, N. S. (1988). The effects of time on the adolescent sibling bereavement process. *Pediatric Nursing, 14,* 333–335.

Hogan, N. S., & Balk, D. E. (1990). Adolescent reactions to sibling death: Perceptions of mothers, fathers, and teenagers. *Nursing Research, 39,* 103–106.

Irving, J. R. (1984). Playing my dead sister's surrogate. *Death Education, 8,* 413–417.

Klyman, C. M. (1986). Pregnancy as a reaction to early childhood sibling loss. *Journal of the American Academy of Psychoanalysis, 14,* 323–335.

Krell, R., & Rabkin, L. (1979). The effects of sibling death on the surviving child: A family perspective. *Family Process, 18,* 471–477.

Martinson, I. M., Davies, E. B., & McClowry, S. G. (1987). The long-term effects of sibling death on self-concept. *Journal of Pediatric Nursing, 2,* 227–235.

McCown, D. E. (1984). Funeral attendance, cremation, and young siblings. *Death Education, 8,* 349–363.

McCown, D. E. (1987). Factors related to bereaved children's behavioral adjustment. In C. Barnes (Ed.), *Recent advances in nursing* (pp. 89–93). London: Churchill Livingstone.

McCown, D. E., & Pratt, C. (1985). Impact of sibling death on children's behavior. *Death Studies, 9,* 323–335.

Michael, S. A. P., & R. G. Lansdown (1986). Adjustment to the death of a sibling. *Archives of Disease in Childhood, 61,* 278–283.

Mufson, T. (1985). Issues surrounding sibling death during adolesence. *Child and Adolescent Social Work, 2,* 204–218.

Pollock, G. H. (1972). Bertha Pappenheim's pathological mourning: Possible effects childhood sibling loss. *Journal of the American Psychiatric Association, 20,* 476–493.

Pollock, G. H. (1973). Bertha Pappenheim: Addenda to her case history. *Journal of the American Psychiatric Association, 21,* 328–332.

Pollock, G. H. (1986). Childhood sibling loss: A family tragedy. *Psychiatric Annals, 16,* 309–314.

Pollock, G. H. (1987). On siblings, childhood sibling loss, and creativity. *Emotions and Behavior Monographs, 4,* 113–167.

Richter, E. (1987). *Losing someone you love: When a brother or sister dies.* New York: Putnam.

Rosen, H. (1985). Prohibitions against mourning in childhood sibling loss. *Omega, 15,* 307–316.

Rosen, H. (1986a). When a sibling dies. *International Journal of Family Psychiatry, 7,* 389–396.

Rosen, H. (1986b). *Unspoken grief: Coping with childhood sibling loss.* New York: Lexington Books.

Rosen, H., & Cohen, H. L. (1981). Children's reactions to sibling loss. *Clinical Social Work Journal, 9,* 211–219.

Schumacher, J. D. (1983). Helping children cope with a sibling's death. In T. T. Frantz & J. C. Hansen (Eds.), *Death in the family.* Rockville, MD: Aspen.

Tooley, K. (1975). The choice of a surviving sibling as the 'scapegoat' in some cases of maternal bereavement. *Journal of Child Psychology and Psychiatry, 16,* 331–339.

Trouy, M. B., & Ward-Larson, C. (1987). Sibling grief. *Neonatal Network, 5,* 35–40.

Widen, H. A. (1987). Phase-specific symptomatic response to sibling loss in late adolescence. *Adolescent Psychiatry, 14,* 218–229.

CHILDREN'S UNDERSTANDING OF DEATH

Childers, P., & Wimmer, M. (1971). The concept of death in early childhood. *Child Development, 42,* 1299–1301.

Fetsch, S. H. (1984). The 7- to 10-year-old child conceptualization of death. *Oncology Nursing Forum, 11,* 52–56.

Grollman, E. A. (1967). *Explaining death to children.* Boston: Beacon.

Grollman, E. A. (1970). *Talking about death: A dialogue between parent and child.* Boston: Beacon.

Kane, B. (1979). Children's concept of death. *Journal of Genetic Psychology, 134,* 141–153.

Koocher, G. P. (1973). Childhood, death and cognitive development. *Developmental Psychology, 9,* 369–375.

Koocher, G. P. (1974). Talking with children about death. *American Journal of Orthopsychiatry, 44,* 404–411.

Lonetto, R. (1980). *Children's conceptions of death.* New York: Springer.

Nagy, M. (1948). The child's theories concerning death. *Journal of Genetic Psychology, 73,* 3–27.

Nagy, M. H. (1959). The child's view of death. In H. Feifel (Ed.), *The meaning of death.* New York: McGraw-Hill.

Reilly, P., Hasazi, J. E., & Bond, L. A. (1983). Children's conceptions of death and personal mortality. *Journal of Pediatric Psychology, 8,* 21–31.

Smilansky, S. (1987). *On death: Helping children understand and cope.* New York: Peter Lang.

Speece, M. W., & Brent, S. B. (1984). Children's understanding of death: A review of three components of a death concept. *Child Development, 55,* 1671–1686.

Tallmer, M., Formanek, R., & Tallmer, J. (1974, Summer). Factors influencing children's concepts of death. *Journal of Clinical Child Psychology,* 17–19.

Wass, H. et al. (1983). Young children's death concepts revisited. *Death Education, 7,* 385–394.

Weber, J. A., & Fournier, D. G. (1986). Death in the family: Children's cognitive understanding and sculptures of family relationship patterns. *Journal of Family Issues, 7,* 277–296.

VIOLENT DEATHS

Black, D., & Kaplan, T. (1988). Father kills mother: Issues and problems encountered by a child psychiatric team. *British Journal of Psychiatry, 153,* 624–630.

Dyregrov, A., & Mitchell, J. T. (1992). Work with traumatized children: Psychological effects and coping strategies. *Journal of Traumatic Stress, 5,* 5–17.

Eth, S., & Pynoos, R. S. (1985). *Post-traumatic stress disorder in children.* Washington, DC: American Psychiatric Press.

Haran, J. (1988). Use of group work to help children cope with the violent death of a classmate. *Social Work with Groups, 11,* 79–92.

Malmquist, C. P. (1986). Children who witness parental murder: Post-traumatic aspects. *Journal American Academy of Child Psychiatry, 25,* 320–325.

McCune, N., & Donnelly, P. (1989). Children surviving parental murder. *British Journal of Psychiatry, 154,* 889.

Nader, K., Pynoos, R., & Fairbanks, L. (1990). Children's PTSD reactions one year after a sniper attack at their school. *American Journal of Psychiatry, 147,* 1526–1530.

Payton, J. B., & Krocker-Tuskan, M. (1988). Children's reactions to loss of parent through violence. *Journal of the American Academy of Child and Adolscent Psychiatry, 27,* 563–566.

Pfeffer, C. R. (1981). Parental suicide: An organizing event in the development of latency age children. *Suicide and Life-Threatening Behavior, 11,* 43–50.

Pynoos, R. S., & Nader, K. (1988). Psychological first aid and treatment approach to children exposed to community violence. *Journal of Traumatic Stress, 1,* 445–472.

Pynoos, R. S., & Nader, K. (1990). Children's exposure to violence and traumatic death. *Psychiatric Annals, 20,* 334–344.

Pynoos, R. S., Nader, K., Fredrick, C., et al. (1987). Grief reactions in school age children following a sniper attack at school. *Israel Journal of Psychiatry and Related Sciences, 24,* 53–56.

Terr, L. C. (1981). Psychic trauma in children: Observations following the Chowchilla school-bus kidnapping. *American Journal of Psychiatry, 138,* 14–19.

Terr, L. C. (1989). Treating psychic trauma in children. *Journal of Traumatic Stress, 2,* 3–20.

References

Achenbach, T. M. (1991). *Manual for the Behavior Checklist/4–18 and 1991 Profile*. Burlington, VT: University of Vermont, Department of Psychiatry.

Achenbach, T. M., & Edelbrock, C. (1983). *Manual for the Child Behavior Checklist and Revised Child Behavior Profile*. Burlington, VT: University of Vermont, Department of Psychiatry.

Altschul, S., & Pollock, G. H. (Eds.). (1988). *Childhood bereavement and its aftermath*. New York: International University Press.

American Psychiatric Association. (1994). *Diagnostic and statistical manual of mental disorders* (4th ed.). Washington, DC: Author.

Baker, J. E., Sedney, M. A., & Gross, E. (1992). Psychological tasks for bereaved children. *American Journal of Orthopsychiatry, 62,* 105–116.

Balk, D. E. (1990). The self-concepts of bereaved adolescents: Silbing death and its aftermath. *Journal of Adolescent Research, 5*(1), 112–132.

Barnes, G. E., & Prosen, H. (1985). Parental death and depression. *Journal of Abnormal Psychology, 94,* 64–69.

Beck, A. T. (1967). *Depression*. New York: Harper & Row.

Bendiksen, R., & Fulton, R. (1975). Childhood bereavement and later behavioral disorders. *Omega, 6,* 45 –60.

Bengesser, G. (1988). Postvention for bereaved family members: Some therapeutic possibilities. *Crisis, 9*(1), 45–48.

Berlinsky, E. B., & Biller, H. B. (1982). *Parental dealth and psychological development*. Lexington, MA: Heath.

Birtchnell, J. (1970a). Early parent death and mental health. *British Journal of Psychiatry, 116,* 281–298.

Birtchnell, J. (1970b). Depression in relation to early and recent parent death. *British Journal of Psychiatry, 116,* 299–305.

Birtchnell, J. (1972). Early parent death and psychiatric diagnosis. *Social Psychiatry, 7,* 202–210.

Birtchnell, J. (1980). Women whose mothers died in childhood: An outcome study. *Psychological Medicine, 10,* 699–713.

Black, D. (1978). The bereaved child. *Journal of Child Psychology and Psychiatry, 19,* 287–292.

Black, D., & Urbanowicz, M. A. (1987). Family intervention with bereaved children. *Journal of Child Psychology and Psychiatry, 28,* 467–476.

Blanck, R., & Blanck, G. (1979). *Ego psychology II.* New York: Columbia University Press.

Bluebond-Langer, M. (1978). *The private worlds of dying children.* Princeton, NJ: Princeton University Press.

Bowen, M. (1978). *Family therapy in clinical practice.* New York: Jason Aronson.

Bowlby, J. (1960). Grief and mourning in infancy and early childhood. *Psychoanalytic Study of the Child, 15,* 9–52.

Bowlby, J. (1963). Pathological mourning and childhood mourning. *Journal of the American Psychoanalytic Association, 11,* 500–541.

Bowlby, J. (1980). *Attachment and loss: Loss, sadness, and depression.* New York: Basic Books.

Bowlby, J. (1982). Attachment and loss: Retrospect and prospect. *American Journal of Orthopsychiatry, 52,* 664–678.

Bowlby-West, L. (1983). The impact of death on the family system. *Journal of Family Therapy, 5,* 279–294.

Breier, A., Kelso, J., Kirwin, P., et al. (1988). Early parental loss and development of adult psychopathology. *Archives of General Psychiatry, 45,* 987–993.

Brisnaire, L., Firestone, P., & Rynord, D. (1990). Factors associated with academic achievement in children following parental separation. *American Journal of Orthopsychiatry, 60,* 67–76.

Brown, F., & Epps, P. (1966). Childhood bereavement and subsequent crime. *British Journal of Psychiatry, 112,* 1043–1048.

Brown, G. W., & Harris, T. O. (1986). Establishing causal links. In H. Katsching (Ed.), *Life events and psychiatric disorders: Controversal issues* (pp. 107–187). Cambridge, UK: Cambridge University Press.

Brown, G. W., Harris, T. O., & Bifulco, A. (1986). Long term effects of early loss of parent. In M. Rutter, C. E. Izard, & P. Read (Eds.), *Depression in young people.* New York: Guilford Press.

Brown, G. W., Harris, L., & Copeland, J. (1977). Depression and loss. *British Journal of Psychiatry, 130,* 1–18.

Buscaglia, L. (1982). *The fall of Freddie the leaf.* Thorofare, NJ: Stack.

Cain, A. C., Fast, I., & Erickson, M. E. (1964). Children's disturbed reactions to the death of a sibling. *American Journal of Orthopsychiatry, 34,* 741–752.

Cook, J. A. (1988). Dad's double binds: Rethinking father's bereavement from a men's studies perspective. *Journal of Contemporary Ethnography, 17,* 285–308.

Coryell, W., Noyes, R., & Clancy, J. (1983). Panic disorder and primary unipolar depression. *Journal of Affective Disorders, 5,* 311–317.

Crook, T., & Raskin, A. (1975). Association of childhood parental loss with attempted suicide and depression. *Journal of Consulting and Clinical Psychology, 43,* 277.

Davies, B. (1987). Family responses to the death of a child: The meaning of memories. *Journal of Palliative Care, 3,* 9–15.

Davies, B. (1988a). Shared life space and sibling bereavement responses. *Cancer Nursing, 11,* 339–347.

Davies, B. (1988b). The family environment in bereaved families and its relationship to surviving sibling behavior. *Children's Health Care, 17,* 22–32.

Davies, B. (1991). Long-term outcomes of adolescent sibling bereavement. *Journal of Adolescent Reserach, 6,* 83–96.

Dennehy, C. (1966). Childhood bereavement and psychiatric illness. *British Journal of Psychiatry, 112,* 1049–1069.

Detmer, C. M., & Lamberti, J. W. (1991). Family grief. *Death Studies, 15,* 363–374.

Deutsch, H. (1937). Absence of grief. *Psychoanalytic Quarterly, 6,* 12–22.

Doherty, W., & Needle, R. (1991). Psychological adjustment and substance use among adolescents before and after a parental divorce. *Child Development, 62,* 328–337.

Dorpat, H., Jackson, J. K., & Ripley, H. S. (1965). Broken homes and attempted and completed suicide. *Archives of General Psychiatry, 12,* 213–216.

Edelman, H. (1994). Motherless daughters: The legacy of loss. New York: Dell.

Elizur, E., & Kaffman, M. (1982). Children's bereavement reactions following death of the father: II. *Journal of the American Academy of Child Psychiatry, 21,* 474–480.

Elizur, E., & Kaffman, M. (1983). Factors influencing the severity of childhood bereavement reactions. *American Journal of Orthopsychiatry, 53,* 668–676.

Fanos, J. H., & Nickerson, B. G. (1991). Long-term effects of sibling death during adolescence. *Journal of Adolescent Research, 6,* 70–82.

Faravelli, C., Webb, T., Ambonetti, A., et al. (1985). Prevalence of traumatic early life events in 31 agoraphobic patients with panic attacks. *American Journal of Psychiatry, 142,* 1493–1494.

Farberow, N., Gallagher, D., Gilewski, M., et al. (1987). An examination of the early impact of bereavement on psychological distress in survivors of suicide. *Gerontologist, 27,* 592–598.

Felner, R. D. et al. (1981). Parental death or divorce and the school adjustment of young children. *American Journal of Community Psychology, 9,* 181–191.

Finkelstein, H. (1988). The long-term effects of early parent death: A reveiw. *Journal of Clinical Psychology, 44,* 3–9.

Fleming, S. J., & Adolph, R. (1986). Helping bereaved adolescents. In C. Corr & J. McNeil (Eds.), *Adolescence and death* (pp. 97–118). New York: Springer.

Forehand, R. (1991). The role of famialy stressors and parent relationships in adolescent functioning. *Journal of the American Academy of Child and Adolescent Psychiatry, 30,* 316–322.

Fox, S. S. (1985). *Good grief: Helping groups of children when a friend dies.* Boston: New England Association for the Education of Young Children.

Fraiberg, S. H. (1959). *The magic years.* New York: Scribners.

Freud, A. (1960). Discussion of Dr. John Bowlby's paper. *Psychoanalytic Study of the Child, 15,* 53–63.

Freud, S. (1917). Mourning and melancholia. In *Standard edition* (Vol. 14). London: Hogarth.

Furman, E. (1974). *A child's parent dies: Studies in childhood bereavement.* New Haven, CT: Yale University Press.

Furman, R. (1964). Death and the young child: Some preliminary considerations. *Psychoanalytic Study of the Child, 19,* 321–333.

Gardner, R. (1983). Children's reactions to parental death. In J. Schowalter et al. (Eds.), *The child and death.* New York: Columbia University Press.

Garmezy, N. (1987). Stress, competence, and development. *American Journal of Orthopsychiatry, 57,* 159–185.

Gelcer, E. (1983). Mourning is a family affair. *Family Process, 22,* 501–516.

Goldney, R. D. (1981). Parental loss and reported childhood stress in young women who attempt suicide. *Acta Psychiatrica Scandinavica, 64,* 34–47.

Granville-Grossman, K. L. (1966). Early bereavement and schizophrenia. *British Journal of Psychiatry, 112,* 465–470.

Gray, R. E. (1989). Adolescents' perceptions of social support after the death of a parent. *Journal of Psychosocial Oncology, 7*(3), 127–144.

Greaves, C. C. (1983). Death in the family: A multifamily therapy approach. *International Journal of Family Psychiatry, 4,* 247–259.

Grollman, E. A. (1967). *Explaining death to children.* Boston: Beacon.

Harris, M. (1995). *The loss that is forever: The lifelong impact of the early death of a mother or father.* New York: Dutton.

Harris, T., Brown, G. W., & Bifulco, A. (1986). Loss of parent in childhood and adult psychiatric disorders: The role of lack of adequate parental care. *Psychological Medicine, 16,* 641–659.

Harter, S. (1979). *Manual: Perceived competence scale for children.* Denver, CO: University of Denver.

Harter, S. (1985). *Processes underlying the construction, maintenance, and enhancement of the self-concept in children.* Hillsdale, NJ: Erlbaum.

Healy, J. M., Stewart, A. J., & Copeland, A. P. (1993). The role of self-blame in children's adjustment to parental separation. *Personality and Social Psychology Bulletin, 19,* 229–289.

Hepworth, J., Ryder, R., & Dreyer, A. (1984). The effect of parental loss on the formation of intimate relationships. *Journal of Marital and Family Therapy, 10,* 73–82.

Hetherington, E. M. (1972). Effects of father absence on personality development in adolescent daughters. *Developmental Psychology, 7,* 313–326.

Hetherington, E. M. (1979). Divorce: A child's perspective. *American Psychologist, 43.*

Hetherington, E. M. (1993). An overview of the Virginia longitudinal study of divorce and remarriage with a focus on early adolescence. *Journal of Family Psychology, 7,* 39–56.

Hill, O. W. (1969). The association of childhood bereavement with suicidal attempts in depressive illness. *British Journal of Psychiatry, 155,* 301–304.

Hogan, N. S. (1988). The effects of time on the adolescent sibling bereavement process. *Pediatric Nursing, 14,* 333–335.

Hoyt, L., Cowen, E., Petro-Carroll, J., et al. (1990). Anxiety and depression in young children of divorce. *Journal of Clinical Child Psychology, 19,* 26–32.

Jacobson, E. (1954). The self and the object world. *Psychoanalytic Study of the Child, 9,* 75–127.

Jewett, C. L. (1982). *Helping children cope with separation and loss.* Cambridge, MA: Harvard Common Press.

Kelly, J. B. (1993). Current research on children's postdivorce adjustment. *Family and Conciliation Courts Review, 31,* 29–49.

Kendler, K. S., Neale, M. D., Kessler, R. C., et al. (1992). Childhood parental loss and adult psychopathology in women: A twin study perspective. *Archives of General Psychiatry, 49,* 109–116.

Klerman, G., & Weissman, M. (1986). The interpersonal approach to understanding depression. In T. Millon & G. Klerman (Eds.), *Contemporary directions in psychopathology.* New York: Guilford Press.

Kliman, G. (Ed.). (1968). *Psychological emergencies in childhood.* New York: Grune & Stratton.

Kranzler, E. M., Shaffer, D., Wasserman, G., et al. (1990). Early childhood bereavement. *Journal of the American Academy of Child and Adolescent Psychiatry, 29,* 513–520.

Krell, R., & Rabkin, L. (1979). The effects of sibling death on the surviving child: A family perspective. *Family Process, 18,* 471–477.

Levi, L., Fales, C., Stein, M., & Sharp, V. (1966). Separation and attempted suicide. *Archives of General Psychiatry, 15,* 158–164.

Lloyd, C. (1980). Life events and depressive disorder reviewed. *Archives of General Psychiatry, 37,* 529–535.

Markusen, E., & Fulton, R. (1971). Childhood bereavement and behavioral disorders: A critical reveiw. *Omega, 2,* 107–117.

Marris, P. (1974). *Loss and change.* London: Routledge & Kegan Paul.

McCown, D. (1987). Factors related to bereaved children's behavioral adjustment. In C. Barnes (Ed.), *Recent advances in nursing* (pp. 89–93). London: Churchill Livingstone.

McCown, D., & Pratt, C. (1985). Impact of sibling death on children's behavior. *Death Studies, 9,* 323–335.

McCubbin, H., Larson, A., & Olson, D. H. (1987). F-COPES: Family crisis oriented personal scales. In H. I. McCubbin & A. Thompson (Eds.), *Family assessment inventories for research and practice.* Madison: University of Wisconsin.

McCubbin, H., Patterson, J., & Wilson, L. (1979). *Family Inventory of Life Events.* St. Paul, MN: University of Minnesota.

McIntyre, B. B. (1990). Art therapy with bereaved youth. *Journal of Palliative Care, 5,* 16–25.

Mireault, G. C., & Bond, L. A. (1992). Parental death in childhood: Perceived vulnerability, and adult depression and anxiety. *American Journal of Orthopsychiatry, 62,* 517–524.

Muir, E., Speirs, A., & Tod, G. (1988). Family intervention and parent involvement in the facilitation of mourning in a 4-year-old boy. *Psychoanalytic Study of the Child, 43,* 367–383.

Mulholland, D., Watt, N., Philpott, A., et al. (1991). Academic performance in children of divorce. *Psychiatry, 54,* 269–280.

Nagy, M. (1948). The child's theories concerning death. *Journal of Genetic Psychology, 73,* 3–27.

Nagy, M. H. (1959). The child's view of death. In H. Feifel (Ed.), *The meaning of death* (pp. 79–98). New York: McGraw-Hill.

Nowicki, S., & Strickland, B. R. (1973). A locus of control scale for children. *Journal of Consulting and Clinical Psychology, 40,* 148–154.

Olson, D. H. (1986). Circumplex model VII: Validation studies and FACES III. *Family Process, 25,* 337–351.

Olson, D. H., Portner, J., & Lavee, Y. (1985). *FACES III*. St. Paul, MN: University of Minnesota Family Social Science.

Oltman, J. E., & Friedman, S. (1965). Report on parental depravation in psychiatric disorder. *Archives of General Psychiatry, 12,* 46–57.

Osterweis, M., Solomon, F., & Greene, M. (Eds.). (1984). *Bereavement: Reactions, consequences, and care.* Washington, DC: National Academy Press.

O'Toole, D., (1989). *Aarvy aardvark finds hope: A read-aloud story for people of all ages.* Burnsville, NC: Mountain Rainbow Press.

Parkes, C. M. (1972). *Bereavement: Studies of grief in adult life.* New York: Intertnational Universities Press.

Paul, N., & Grosser, G. H. (1965). Operational mourning and its role in conjoint family therapy. *Community Mental Health Journal, 1,* 339–345.

Perloff, L., & Fetzer, B. (1986). Self–other judgments and perceived vulnerability to victimization. *Journal of Personality and Social Psychology, 50,* 502–510.

Piaget, J. (1954). *The construction of reality in the child* (M. Cook, Trans.). New York: Basic Books.

Portes, P. R. et al. (1992). Family functions and children's post divorce adjustment. *American Journal of Orthopsychiatry, 62,* 613–617.

Radloff, L. (1977). The CES-D scale: A self-report depression scale for research in the general population. *Applied Psychological Measurement, 1,* 385–401.

Radloff, L., & Teri, L. (1986). Use of the Center for Epidemiological Studies Depression Scale with older adults. *Clinical Gerontologist, 5,* 116–136.

Raphael, B. (1983). *The anatomy of bereavement.* New York: Basic Books.

Raskin, M., Peeke, H., Dickman, W., et al. (1982). Panic and generalized anxiety disorders: Developmental antecedents and precipitants. *Archives of General Psychiatry, 39,* 687–689.

Reese, M. F. (1982). Growing up: The impact of loss and change. In D. Belle (Ed.), *Lives in stress: Women and depression* (pp. 65–88). Beverly Hills, CA: Sage.

Rosen, H. (1985). Prohibitions against mourning in childhood sibling loss. *Omega, 15,* 307–316.

Rosen, H., & Cohen, H. L. (1981). Children's reactions to sibling loss. *Clinical Social Work Journal, 9,* 211–219.

Rosenblatt, P., & Elde, C. (1990). Shared reminiscence about a deceased parent: Implications for grief education and grief counseling. *Family Relations, 39,* 206–210.

Rosenthal, P. A. (1980). Short-term family therapy and pathological grief resolution with children and adolescents. *Family Process, 19,*151–159.

Rutter, M. (1984). Psychopathology and development. *Australia and New Zealand Journal of Psychiatry, 18,* 225–234.

Sanders, C. M. (1979–1980). A comparison of adult bereavement in the death of a spouse, child, and parent. *Omega, 10,* 303–322.

Schwartz-Borden, G. (1986). Grief work: Prevention and intervention. *Social Casework,* 499–505.

Segal, R. M. (1984). Helping children express grief through symbolic communication. *Social Casework, 65,* 590–599.

Seligman, R., Gleser, G., & Raugh, J. (1974). The effects of earlier parental loss in adolescence. *Archives of General Psychiatry, 31,* 475–479.

Shaw, D., Emery, R., Tver, M. (1993). Parental functioning and children's adjustment in families of divorce. *Journal of Abnormal Child Psychology, 21,* 119–134.

Shuchter, S. R., & Zisook, S. (1986). Treatment of spousal bereavement: A multidimensional approach. *Psychiatric Annals, 16,* 295–305.

Siegel, K., Mesagno, F. P., & Christ, G. (1990). A prevention program for bereaved children. *American Journal of Orthopsychiatry, 60,* 168–175.

Sills, C., Clarkson, P., & Evans, R. (1988). Systemic integrative psychotherapy with a young bereaved girl. *Transactional Analysis Journal, 18,* 102–109.

Silverman, P. R. (1986). *Widow to widow.* New York: Springer.

Silverman, P. R. (1989). The impact of parental death on college-age women. *Psychiatric Clinics of North America, 10,* 387–404.

Silverman, P. R., Nickman, S., & Worden, J. W. (1992). Detachment revisited: The child's reconstruction of a dead parent. *American Journal of Orthopsychiatry, 62,* 494–503.

Silverman, P. R., & Worden, J. W. (1992). Children's reactions in the early months after the death of a parent. *American Journal of Orthopsychiatry, 62,* 93–104.

Smilansky, S. (1987). *On death: Helping children understand and cope.* New York: Peter Lang.

Smith, I. (1991). Preschool children play out their grief. *Death Studies, 15,* 169–176.

Sood, B., Weller, E., Weller, R., et al. (1992). Somatic complaints in grieving children. *Comprehensive Mental Health Care, 2,* 17–25.

Spinetta, J. J., & Deasey-Spinetta, P. (Eds.). (1981). *Living with childhood cancer.* St. Louis, MN: Mosby.

Strength, J. M. (1991). Factors influencing the mother–child relationship following the death of the father. *Dissertation Abstracts International, 52,* 3310B.

Tennant, C. (1988). Parental loss in childhood: Its effect in adult life. *Archives of General Psychiatry, 45,* 1045–1049.

Tennant, C., Bebbington, P., & Hurry, J. (1980). Parent death in childhood and risk of adult depressive disorders: A review. *Psychological Medicine, 10,* 289–299.

Tennant, C., Bebbington, P., & Hurry, J. (1981). Parental loss in childhood: Relationship to adult psychiatric impairment and contact with psychiatric services. *Archives of General Psychiatry, 38,* 309–314.

Tooley, K. (1975). The choice of a surviving sibling as the 'scapegoat' in some cases of maternal bereavement. *Journal of Child Psychology and Psychiatry, 16,* 331–339.

Torgersen, S. (1986). Childhood and family characteristics in panic and generalized anxiety disorders. *American Journal of Psychiatry, 143,* 630–632.

Tweed, J., Schoenbach, V., George, L., et al. (1989). The effect of childhood parental death and divorce on six-month history of anxiety disorders. *British Journal of Psychiatry, 154,* 823–828.

Vaillant, G. E. (1985). Loss as a metaphor for attachment. *American Journal of Psychoanalysis, 42,* 59–67.

Van Eerdewegh, M., Bieri, M., Parilla, R. H., et al. (1982). The bereaved child. *British Journal of Psychiatry, 140,* 23–29.

Van Eerdewegh, M. M., Clayton, P. J., & Van Eerdewegh, P. (1985). The bereaved child: Variables influencing early psychopathology. *British Journal of Psychiatry, 14,* 188–194.

Volkan, V. D. (1981). *Linking objects and linking phenomena.* New York: International Universities Press.

Wallerstein, J. S., & Blakeslee, S. (1989). *Second chances: Men, women, and children a decade after divorce.* New York: Ticknor & Fields.

Wallerstein, J. S. (1991). The long-term effects of divorce on children: A review. *Journal of the American Academy of Child and Adolescent Psychiatry, 30.*

Warmbrod, M. E. T. (1986). Counseling bereaved children: Stages in the process. *Social Casework,* 351–358.

Wass, H., & Corr, C. (1982). *Helping children copy with death.* Washington, DC: Hemisphere. (Second edition published 1984)

Watt, N. F., & Nicholi, A. (1979). Early death of a parent as an etiological factor in schizophrenia. *American Journal of Orthopsychiatry, 49,* 465–473.

Webb, N. B. (Ed.). (1993). *Helping bereaved children: A handbook for practitioners.* New York: Guilford Press.

Weisman, A. D. (1972). *On dying and denying.* New York: Behavioral Publications.

Wilson, I. C., Altop, L., & Buffaloe, W. J. (1967). Parental bereavement in childhood: MMPI profiles in a depressed population. *British Journal of Psychiatry, 113,* 761–764.

Winnicott, D. W. (1953). Transitional objects and transitional phenomena. *International Journal of Psycho-Analysis, 34,* 89–97.

Wolfelt, A. D. (1993). The misdiagnosis of ADHD in bereaved children. *The Forum Newsletter, 19,* 9–10, 18.

Wolfelt, A. D. (1996). *Healing the bereaved child.* Ft. Collins, CO: Companion.

Wolfenstein, M. (1966). How is mourning possible? *Psychoanalytic Study of the Child, 21,* 93–123.

Worden, J. W. (1976). *Personal death awareness.* Englewood Cliffs, NJ: Prentice Hall.

Worden, J. W. (1982). *Grief counseling and grief therapy: A handbook for the mental health practitioner* (1st ed.). New York: Springer.

Worden, J. W. (1991). *Grief counseling and grief therapy: A handbook for the mental health practitioner* (2nd ed.). New York: Springer.

Worden, J. W., & Monahan, J. (1993). Bereaved parents. In A. Armstrong-Dailey & S. Goltzer (Eds.), *Hospice care for children* (pp. 122–139). Oxford: Oxford University Press.

Worden, J. W., & Silverman, P. R. (1993). Grief and depression in newly widowed parents with school-age children. *Omega, 27*(3), 251–260.

York, J. B., & Weinstein, S. A. (1980–1981). The effect of a videotape about death on bereaved children in family therapy. *Omega, 11,* 355–361.

Zambelli, G. C., Clark, E., Baile, L., et al. (1988). An interdisciplinary approach to clinical intervention for childhood bereavement. *Death Studies, 12,* 41–50.

Zambelli, G. C., & DeRosa, A. P. (1992). Bereavement support groups for school-age children: Theory, intervention, and case example. *American Journal of Orthopsychiatry, 62,* 484–493.

Zilberg, N. J., Weiss, D. S., & Horowitz, M. J. (1982). Impact of events scale: A cross-validation study. *Journal of Consulting and Clinical Psychology, 50,* 407–414.

Author Index

Achenbach, T. M., 5, 97, 173, 179, *203*
Adams-Greenly, M., *192*
Adolph, R., 88, 90, *204*
Agee, J., *191*
Albert, R. S., *185*
Althous, M., *183*
Altop, L., *196, 210*
Altschul, S., 155, 159, *183, 201*
Ambonetti, A., *195, 203*
American Psychiatric Association., 150, *201*
Ankenbauer, M. R., *197*
Anthony, S., *183*
Archer, D. N., *191*
Arthur, B., *183*

B

Baile, L., *210*
Baker, J. E., 2, 12, *183, 201*
Balk, D. E., 154, *188, 197, 201*
Barnes, G. E., 105, *194, 201*
Beard, P., *183*
Bebbington, P., *196, 209*
Beck, A. T., 154, *201*
Becker, D., *183*
Becker, J., *189*
Bemporad, J. R., *188*
Bendiksen, R., 107, *195, 201*
Bengesser, G., 155, *191, 201*

Bentovim, A., *183*
Berden, G., *183*
Berlinsky, E. B., 68, 91, 92, 100, 160, *186, 201*
Berman, D., *187*
Berman, H., *188*
Bertman, S., *192*
Bieri, M., *187, 207*
Bifulco, A., *195, 196, 202, 205*
Biller, H. B., 68, 91, 92, 100, 160, *186, 201*
Birenbaum, L. K., *197*
Birtchnell, J., 106, 107, *195, 201, 202*
Black, D., 62, 157, 159, *183, 191, 200, 202*
Blakeslee, S., 126, 128, 129, *190, 209*
Blanck, G., 79, *202*
Blanck, R., 79, *202*
Blinder, B., *197*
Bluebond-Langer, M., 11, *202*
Bond, L. A., 109, *187, 199, 206*
Bowen, M., 130, 158, *202*
Bowes, J. M., *187*
Bowlby, J., 9, 108, 109, 141, *183, 195, 202*
Bowlby-West, L., 157, *191, 202*
Braver, S., *189, 190*
Breier, A., 108, 109, *195, 202*
Brent, S. B., *199*
Bright, P. D., *188*
Brisnaire, L., 133, *202*

Subject Index